J R Simpson

A PAEDIATRIC VADE-MECUM

A Paediatric Vade-Mecum

EDITED BY

JACK INSLEY

M.B., F.R.C.P.E., D.C.H.

*Consultant Paediatrician and Clinical Geneticist,
Birmingham Area Health Authority (Teaching)*

and

BEN WOOD

D.M., F.R.C.P., D.C.H.

*Tenth Edition
(Reprint)*

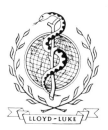

LLOYD-LUKE (MEDICAL BOOKS) LTD
49 NEWMAN STREET
LONDON
1984

First six editions published by the
United Birmingham Hospitals

SEVENTH EDITION .	.	.	.	. 1970
Italian Translation	.	.	.	. 1971
Reprinted .	.	.	.	. 1972
French Translation	.	.	.	. 1973
EIGHTH EDITION .	.	.	.	. 1974
Greek Translation .	.	.	.	. 1976
NINTH EDITION	.	.	.	. 1977
TENTH EDITION .	.	.	.	. 1982
Reprinted .	.	.	.	. 1984

FILMSET, PRINTED AND BOUND IN ENGLAND BY
HAZELL WATSON AND VINEY LIMITED,
MEMBER OF THE BPCC GROUP,
AYLESBURY, BUCKS

ISBN 0 85324 158 9

CONTRIBUTORS

D. C. A. CANDY, M.B., B.S., M.SC., M.R.C.P.

M. JOYCE CARLYLE, B.SC., M.D.

NEETA M. DAIN, B.PHARM., M.P.S.

ANNE DE LOOY, B.SC., PH.D., S.R.D.

G. M. DURBIN, B.M., B.CH., M.R.C.P.

R. H. GEORGE, M.B., CH.B., M.R.C.PATH.

K. D. GRIFFITHS, B.SC., PH.D.

F. G. H. HILL, M.B., CH.B., M.R.C.PATH.

A. D. HOCKLEY, M.B., B.S., F.R.C.S.E.

C. A. HUGHES, M.B., B.S., M.SC., M.R.C.P., D.C.H.

D. McG. JACKSON, M.D., F.R.C.S.

P. M. JEAVONS, F.R.C.P., F.R.C.PSYCH.

JILLIAN R. MANN, M.B., B.S., M.R.C.P., D.C.H.

M. PANTER-BRICK, M.B., CH.B., M.R.C.P., D.C.H.

P. H. W. RAYNER, M.B., CH.B., F.R.C.P.

B. T. RUDD, B.SC., PH.D.

G. W. RYLANCE, M.B., CH.B., M.R.C.P.

E. D. SILOVE, M.D., F.R.C.P., F.R.C.P.E.

MARGARET A. TONGUE, M.B., CH.B.

J. E. S. VARLEY, F.R.C.P., F.R.C.PSYCH., D.P.M.

P. H. WELLER, M.B., B.CHIR., M.R.C.P.

B. A. WHARTON, M.D., F.R.C.P., D.C.H.

R. H. R. WHITE, M.D., F.R.C.P., D.C.H.

M. H. WINTERBORN, M.B., B.S., F.R.C.P.

FOREWORD

It is an honour and a pleasure to have been asked to write this foreword. I follow in the distinguished footsteps of the late Sir Douglas Hubble who, in addition to writing the foreword for the previous three editions, made important contributions to the success of *The Vade Mecum of the Birmingham Children's Hospital*. It was he who persuaded Dr. Ben Wood to accept the editorship of the fifth and subsequent editions, and proposed in 1970 that the responsibility for producing the *Vade Mecum* should be transferred from private hands to professional publishers. The combined results has been a publication of consistently high standard, appreciated by an ever widening readership.

Dr. Jack Insley has taken on this tenth edition aided by Dr. Wood as co-editor. Their combined editorial skills have produced a volume which meets two apparently incompatible objectives. It contains a wealth of data and much practical advice and guidance on the investigation and management of common paediatric conditions, while remaining genuinely pocket-sized. The contents are clear, concise, up-to-date and, above all, useful.

Prefaces to earlier editions of the *Vade Mecum* appeared to indicate that the book was designed mainly for junior doctors. Personal observation and, indeed, experience leave me in no doubt that the *Vade Mecum* is essential reading for consultants as well. The editors have acknowledged this trend by including, for example, an expanded section on paediatric emergencies and a new chapter on the practical complexities of total parenteral nutrition.

All who have come to rely on the *Vade Mecum* will be quick to purchase this latest edition. In addition, I am confident that this volume will find new friends and admirers. The editors should already be looking forward to the next edition.

ALEXANDER S. McNEISH
Leonard Parsons Professor of Paediatrics
and Child Health, University of Birmingham

EDITORS' NOTE

We have taken the opportunity in this edition to seek help in the revision of practically the whole book. The result is a bulkier pocketful but some of the data cannot at present be found elsewhere. The chapter on primary care introduces the junior to some commoner problems which he may be asked to deal with in the Casualty Department or in Out-Patients. Other additions include a section on parenteral nutrition. The chapter on the newborn has been rewritten; the section on paediatric emergencies expanded; while that on development now embraces the Denver developmental scoring test.

Many new contributors have been added to the list on page v and are identified by initials at the end of their sections. We are also extremely grateful for advice from Sean Corkery, John Gowar, Michael Tarlow and the late Noel Raine. There are only three authors who are no longer working in, or attached to, the Children's Hospital: Miss Anne de Looy, now lecturer in dietetics in the University of Leeds; Mr. Douglas Jackson, now retired from the Birmingham Accident Hospital, and Professor Peter Jeavons of Aston University.

The text rarely comments on the timing of decisions when dealing with ill patients, such as "calling in" the surgeon or transferring to another unit. We now take the opportunity of reminding colleagues that whenever possible such decisions should be made early in the day. The five o'clock on Friday afternoon syndrome is bad for everyone, particularly the patient.

All reasonable steps have been taken to ensure accuracy of data on dosages, normal values and levels. Although press proofs were checked most carefully we cannot accept responsibility for printing errors and we recommend the golden rule that if in doubt consult the pharmacist.

September 1981

JACK INSLEY
BEN WOOD

CONTENTS

I

GROWTH, DEVELOPMENT
AND
OTHER NORMAL DATA

PHYSICAL GROWTH

The tables for weight, height and skull circumference give an indication of the percentile status at the time of examination; for long-term observation of the individual child suitable charts are available as shown below.

CENTILE TABLE FOR GIRLS

Gestation weeks	Weight kg			Height cm*			Skull Circumference cm*		
	10	50	90	10	50	90	10	50	90
28	0·75	1·1	1·5	36·5	38	40	25	26	27·5
30	1·0	1·5	2·1	38·5	40·5	42	27	28	29·5
32	1·5	2·0	2·7	41	43	44·5	28·5	30	31
34	1·8	2·5	3·3	43	45	47	30	31·5	33
36	2·3	2·8	3·6	45	47	49	31·5	33	34
38	2·6	3·2	3·8	47	48·5	51	32·5	34	35·5
40	2·8	3·4	4·0	48	49	52	33·5	35	36

Age	3	50	97	3	50	97	3	50	97
3 months	4·2	5·2	7·0	55	58	62	37	40	43
6 months	5·9	7·3	9·4	61	65	69	40	43	45
9 months	7·0	8·7	10·9	65	70	74	42	44	47
12 months	7·6	9·6	12·0	69	74	78	43	46	48
18 months	8·8	10·9	13·6	75	80	85	45	47	50
2 years	9·6	12·0	14·9	79	85	91	46	48	51
3 years	11·2	14·1	17·4	86	93	100	47	49	52
4 years	13	16	20	92	100	109			
5 years	15	18	23	98	107	116	48	50	53
6 years	16	20	27	104	114	123			
7 years	18	23	30	109	120	130			
8 years	19	25	35	114	125	136	50	52	54
9 years	21	28	40	120	130	142			
10 years	23	31	48	125	136	148			
11 years	25	35	56	130	143	155			
12 years	28	40	64	135	149	164	51	53	56
13 years	32	46	70	142	156	168			
14 years	37	51	73	148	160	172	52	54	57
15 years	42	54	74	150	162	173			
16 years	45	56	75	151	162	174			
17 years	46	56	75	—	—	—			
18 years	46	57	75	—	—	—			

* To nearest half cm.

From Gairdner, D., and Pearson, J. (1971), *Arch. Dis. Childh.*, **46,** 783; and Tanner, J. M., Whitehouse, R. H., and Takaishi, M. (1966) *Arch. Dis. Childh.*, **41,** 454.

Adapted from Westrop, C. K., and Barber, C. R. (1956), *J. Neurol., Neurosurg. Psychiat.*, **19,** 52.

CENTILE TABLE FOR BOYS

Gestation weeks	Weight kg			Height cm*			Skull Circumference cm*		
	10	50	90	10	50	90	10	50	90
28	0·8	1·1	1·4	36	38	40	25	26	27·5
30	1·1	1·5	2·0	38·5	40·5	42	27	28	29·5
32	1·5	2·0	2·6	41	43	44·5	28·5	30	31
34	2·0	2·5	3·2	43	45	47	30	31·5	33
36	2·4	3·0	3·6	45	47	49	31·5	33	34
38	2·6	3·3	3·9	47	48·5	51	32·5	34	35·5
40	2·9	3·5	4·2	48	50	53	33·5	35	36·5
Age	3	50	97	3	50	97	3	50	97
3 months	4·4	5·7	7·2	55	60	65	38	41	43
6 months	6·2	7·8	9·8	62	66·5	71	41	44	46
9 months	7·6	9·3	11·6	66·5	71	76	43	46	47
12 months	8·4	10·3	12·8	70	75	80	44	47	49
18 months	9·4	11·7	14·2	75	81	87	46	49	51
2 years	10·2	12·7	15·7	80	87	93	47	50	52
3 years	11·6	14·7	17·8	86	95	102	48	50	53
4 years	13	15	21	94	101	110			
5 years	14	19	23	100	108	117	49	51	54
6 years	16	21	27	105	114	124			
7 years	17	23	30	110	120	130			
8 years	19	25	34	115	126	137	50	52	55
9 years	21	27·5	39	120	132	143			
10 years	23	30	44	125	137	148			
11 years	25	34	50	129	142	154			
12 years	27	38	58	133	147	160	51	54	56
13 years	30	43	64	138	153	168			
14 years	33	49	71	144	160	176	53	56	58
15 years	39	55	76	152	167	182			
16 years	46	60	79	158	172	185			
17 years	49	62	80	162	174	187			
18 years	50	64	82	162	175	187			

* To nearest half cm.

CHARTS

Weight, length, head circumference charts from 28 weeks gestation to 100 weeks by Gairdner, D., and Pearson, J. Printed by Creasey's Ltd., Castlemead, Hereford SG14 1LH.

Growth and Development record, by Tanner, J. M., and Whitehouse, R. H. Printed by Printwell Press Ltd., Bristow Works, Bristow Road, Hounslow, Middlesex.

DEVELOPMENT

The development of their children is of great concern to most parents, and enquiry into the history of past and present achievements is central to developmental assessment. A few guidelines are given here, a table of limit ages for key abilities and then the Denver developmental screening test. The test was standardised on an American and British population which included 12 per cent non-Caucasian children. Some warning signs from the history and physical examination follow.

It is assumed that the conventional medical history and detailed physical examination will be performed; these additional signs are given to alert the enquirer to areas of particular concern for developmental problems. Common misconceptions are given, and then several references to normal and abnormal development.

General Guidelines to Development Assessment

Conduct the examination with the child dressed and comfortable, before any physical examination. Stay ahead of the child, who will easily become bored. Observe his visual, vocal and auditory ability as you take the history and play with him. Congratulate the child for every effort and don't allow his mother to criticise him while he is working with you or with her.

Take a thorough history of the child's development, his relationships and his environment, as well as medical events. Allow fully for prematurity. Beware of assessing a child who is hungry, tired, ill, has had a recent seizure or a child whose mother is upset. Enquire precisely into the mother's concern.

Look for behavioural qualities of alertness, a glint in the eye, rapidity of response, interest in examiner, in surroundings and events, degree of determination, persistence and concentration.

Record all your observations for comparison later on. Interpret your findings in the light of the history and accompanying physical and neurological information, using common sense and caution. Repeated examinations are often necessary and worthwhile, particularly to judge *rate* of progress. Wrong diagnoses do great harm. Say nothing until certain. Fifteen per cent of children will have a developmental problem, 2 per cent will have a severe problem.

LIMIT AGES FOR KEY ABILITIES

This is the age in months by which time all children should show this ability. Full allowance must be made for prematurity. Further examination is indicated if a child of given age does not show this ability. The average child will have achieved the ability long before the limit age.

Age in Months	Ability
1	Some indication of attention.
2	Visual attention to faces and objects. Some response to nearby voices and everyday noises.
3	Head held erect when vertical. Smiles at mother.
4	Hand relaxed, not fisted. Interest shown in people and playthings.
5	Reaches for object. No head lag.
6	Asymmetric tonic neck reflex absent. Visual fixation and following established.
7	Holds objects in both hands.
10	Sits independently on firm surface. Uses tuneful babble. Bears most of weight on legs. Chews lumpy food.
12	Attends to specific words—(No, Dad, Baby). Index finger approach.
15	Releases held object.
18	Walks alone, has stopped casting, mouthing and drooling.
21	Kicks a ball. Says single words with meaning.
27	Puts 2–3 words together into a phrase.
36	Stands on each leg 1–2 seconds. Talks in sentences.
48	Uses fully intelligible speech.

RAPID DEVELOPMENT ASSESSMENT AT FIXED AGES

A rapid developmental check is used in follow-up clinics attached to neonatal units when appointments are made at 6 and 12 months and when appropriate at 18 and 24 months.

Remember to allow for gestational age when such appointments are made.

The following steps have usually been achieved by the time the infant reaches 6, 12, 18 and 24 months. If obvious discrepancies are apparent proceed to full Denver developmental score and determine whether delay is global or partial suggesting a specific motor, visual, auditory or social deficit.

6 Months

Rises on to wrists; rolls from back to front; sits with support, head erect and back straight; bears weight on feet.

Turns head to person talking.

Whole hand grasp—often both hands; all objects to mouth; fixes small objects within 6–12 inches; takes small cube from table.

Babbles or coos to voice or music.

12 Months

Walks, one or both hands held; walks or sidesteps around pen; pivots when sitting; drinks from cup with a little assistance; helps with dressing by holding out arm or foot; demonstrates affection to familiars.

Knows and immediately turns to own name.

Babbles incessantly in "conversational cadences"; comprehends simple instructions associated with gesture, e.g. "give it to . . .", "come to . . .".

Picks up fine objects with neat pincer grasp; drops and throws toys and watches them fall to the ground; explores small model car.

18 Months

Climbs on to chair and then sits; walks upstairs with helping hand, creeps downstairs. Drinks from cup held with both hands; takes off shoes and socks; puts small objects in and out of containers.

Says 6–20 recognisable words and understands many more; hands over named objects; enjoys rhymes and tries to join in.

Builds 3-cube tower after demonstration; turns pages several at a time; picks up small objects delicately on sight.

2 Years

Walks up and down steps; runs safely; squats to play with toys on ground; climbs on to furniture to open doors.

Asks for food and drink; follows mother and simultaneously imitates domestic activity in play; constantly demanding mother's attention.

Shows correctly and repeats on request words for four parts of the body; uses about 50 words; two-word phrases.

Removes paper wrapping from small sweet; holds pencil using thumb and two fingers; makes circular scribble, as well as to and fro and dots; hand preference usually obvious; turns single pages.

The Denver Developmental Screening Test

Standard Test Materials

Red wool ball, raisins, rattle with narrow handle, 1-inch square blocks (2 red, 2 blue, 2 yellow, 2 green), small clear glass bottle with ⅝-inch opening, small bell, tennis ball, pencil, 8 inch × 11 inch plain unlined paper.

Directions

1. The full screening test will take 15–20 minutes in good conditions and is detailed in the *Journal of Pediatrics* for 1967.* The abbreviated text is set out below. The footnote numbers refer to the numbers on the Denver bar chart, and the notes explain how each test is done.

2. Make child and parent comfortable with chair and working table appropriate to child's size, in a non-distracting, quiet room. Child may sit in parent's lap.

3. Explain to parent that child will *not* be expected to do everything asked of him.

4. Draw vertical line on the form through child's chronological age (C.A.) subtracting weeks of gestation below 40. Note today's date and tester's identity at top of line.

5. Work through the test from top to bottom starting well below C.A., and working through C.A. to point of failure. Start with items which can be passed by report (R on scoring sheet). If parent says child can do item, but you are unable to get him to, certain items marked R may be "passed" by report. Items may be given in any order, but the order from younger to older, top to bottom has proved easiest. *Three trials* at each item, except where otherwise specified, are

* Frankenburg, W. K. and Dodds, J. B. (1967) The Denver Developmental Screening Test. *J. Pediat.*, **71**, 181–191.

allowed, before failure is recorded. Praise the child for all efforts, whether or not he succeeds. Remove all test materials except the one being used.

6. Mark the bars P—Pass, F—Fail, R—Refusal, N.O.—No opportunity (based on history). Join highest passes in each category for profile.

7. Apart from these specific tests, the tester should also record general observations (how the child feels at the time of the test, relation to the tester, attention span, verbal behaviour, self-confidence, etc.).

Interpretation of Results

The DDST is interpreted as **Normal, Questionable, Abnormal** and **Untestable** based on the number of delays on each test. To interpret the results of a test properly, follow the steps listed below, remembering that a delay is any failure which falls completely to the left of the age line:

Step 1. Mark each delay by heavily shading the right end of the bar

Step 2. Count the sectors which have 2 or more delays

Step 3. Count the sectors which have 1 delay and no passes intersecting the age line in that same sector.

Step 4. Use the formula shown below to interpret the results.

Abnormal
OR
2 or more sectors with 2 or more delays
2 or more delays in a sector *plus* 1 or more other sectors with 1 delay and no passes intersecting the age line *in that same sector*.

Questionable
OR
1 sector with 2 or more delays
1 delay in 1 or more sectors without any passes intersecting the age line *in that same sector*.

Untestable
when REFUSALS occur in numbers large enough to cause the test result to be QUESTIONABLE or ABNORMAL *if* they were scored as failures.

Normal
any condition not listed above.

DENVER DEVELOPMENTAL SCREENING TEST

(Numbers refer to the numbers on the DDST following, and the notes explain how each test is done.)

1. Try to get child to smile by smiling, talking or waving to him. Do not touch him.
2. When child is playing with toy, pull it away from him. Pass if he resists.
3. Child does not have to be able to tie shoes or button in the back.
4. Move yarn slowly in an arc from one side to the other, about 6 inches above child's face.
   Pass if eyes follow 90° to midline. (Past midline; 180°)
5. Pass if child grasps rattle when it is touched to the backs or tips of fingers.
6. Pass if child continues to look where yarn disappeared or tries to see where it went. Yarn should be dropped quickly from sight from tester's hand without arm movement.
7. Pass if child picks up raisin with any part of thumb and a finger.
8. Pass if child picks up raisin with the ends of thumb and index finger using an overhand approach.

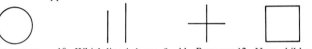

9. Pass any enclosed form. Fail continuous round motions.
10. Which line is longer? (Not bigger.) Turn paper upside down and repeat. (3/3 or 5/6)
11. Pass any crossing lines.
12. Have child copy first. If failed, demonstrate.

When giving items 9, 11 and 12, do not name the forms. Do not demonstrate 9 and 11.

13. When scoring, each pair (2 arms, 2 legs, etc.) counts as one part.
14. Point to picture and have child name it. (No credit is given for sounds only.)

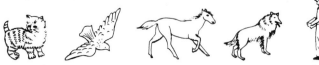

15. Tell child to: Give block to Mummy; put block on table; put block on floor. Pass 2 of 3. (Do not help child by pointing, moving head or eyes.)
16. Ask child: What do you do when you are cold? . . . hungry? . . . tired? Pass 2 of 3.
17. Tell child to: Put block *on* table; *under* table; *in front* of chair, *behind* chair. Pass 3 of 4. (Do not help child by pointing, moving head or eyes.)
18. Ask child: If fire is hot, ice is ?; Mother is a woman, Dad is a ?; a horse is big, a mouse is ?. Pass 2 of 3.
19. Ask child: What is a ball? . . . lake? . . . desk? . . . house? . . . banana? . . . curtain? . . . ceiling? . . . hedge? . . . pavement? Pass if defined in terms of use, shape, what it is made of or general category (such as banana is fruit, not just yellow). Pass 6 of 9.

20. Ask child: What is a spoon made of? . . . a shoe made of? . . . a door made of? (No other objects may be substituted.) Pass 3 of 3.
21. When placed on stomach, child lifts chest off table with support of forearms and/or hands.
22. When child is on back, grasp his hands and pull him to sitting. Pass if head does not hang back.
23. Child may use wall or rail only, not person. May not crawl.
24. Child must throw ball overhand 3 feet to within arm's reach of tester.
25. Child must perform standing broad jump over width of test sheet. (8½ inches)
26. Tell child to walk forward, ⊂⊃ ⊂⊃ ⊂⊃ ⊂⊃ → heel within 1 inch of toe. Tester may demonstrate. Child must walk 4 consecutive steps, 2 out of 3 trials.
27. Bounce ball to child who should stand 3 feet away from tester. Child must catch ball with hands, not arms, 2 out of 3 trials.
28. Tell child to walk backward, ← ⊂⊃ ⊂⊃ ⊂⊃ ⊂⊃ toe within 1 inch of heel. Tester may demonstrate. Child must walk 4 consecutive steps, 2 out of 3 trials.

Warning Signs from Parental History for Developmental Problems

Non-attendance, unless due to child or parent being ill, may be an indication of an at-risk family.

Maternal anxiety, depression or passivity. Mother's observations should be explored seriously and thoroughly.

Feeding problems, apathy, irritability, head-banging, cot-rocking or hostility in an infant.

A toddler who is too good, has a flat toneless voice, repeats rituals or is obsessive, has night terrors or excessive tantrums.

A toddler who is over-friendly or withdrawn, wet by day, who soils, sucks his thumb excessively or is unable to leave his mother.

Warning Signs in Physical Examination for Developmental Problems

At any age: apathy, inactivity, head size out of proportion to length or crossing centile lines (too large or too small), abnormal rates of growth in weight and height, congenital anomalies, including cleft palate, colobomata of the eye, cataract, optic atrophy, deformity of the external ear, odd facies, congenital heart disease, symmetrical defects of hands and feet, unusual hair and hairline.

Six months: squint, nystagmus, persistent hand regard or fisting, preference for one hand, adductor tone at hip, limited abduction in flexion at hip.

DENVER DEVELOPMENTAL SCREENING TEST ©1969 William K. Frankenberg, M.D., and Josiah B. Dodds, Ph.D.
University of Colorado Medical Centre

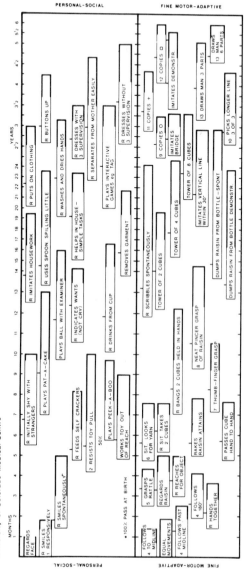

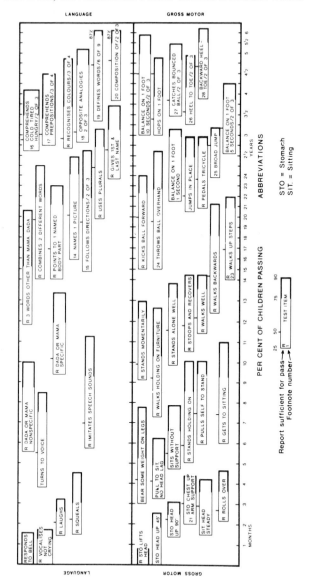

PER CENT OF CHILDREN PASSING

ABBREVIATIONS

STO = Stomach
SIT = Sitting

Ten months: Absence of chewing, no sound localisation, lack of eye-to-eye regard, squint, inability to follow and search for fallen toy, ataxic reach and grasp, unwillingness to bear weight, persistent neonatal reflexes.

Eighteen months: Lack of vocalisation, persistent mouthing of toys and drooling, apparent deafness and lack of visual interest, abnormal grasp, asymmetrical hand use or posture, inability to stand alone.

Two years: Lack of recognisable words, apparent deafness, visual disinterest, unfocused play, inability to walk free, asymmetrical movement, tone or posture.

Three years: Not putting phrases together, deafness, refractive error, abnormal posture, gait, tone or hand use, signs of tuberous sclerosis including adenoma sebaceum, shagreen patches and retinal phakoma.

Four years: Inability to converse with examiner, unfocused or obsessional activity.

Common Misconceptions about Child Development

That ESN parents will necessarily have a child of low intelligence.

That a retarded child who plays with one toy for hours on end is showing good concentration.

That a good-looking, co-operative, well-behaved child is mentally superior.

That ugly, congenitally malformed, lazy, blind or deaf babies are mentally slow.

That hearing cannot be assessed before or independently of vision in a baby under one year.

That development proceeds steadily and evenly in any child.

That there is truly an average child.

M.J.C.

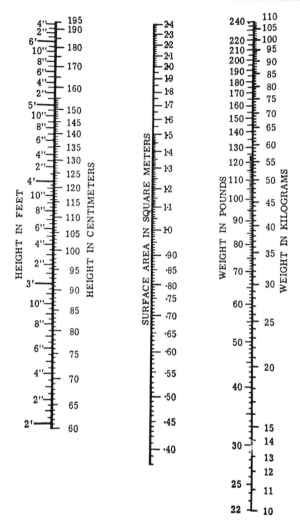

Surface area nomogram. (Adapted from J. R. Geigy, S.A., data.)

CHRONOLOGICAL ORDER OF APPEARANCE OF OSSEOUS CENTRES

	BIRTH	1 YEAR	2	3	4	5
Shoulder 0	Head of humerus (3 *mths.*)	Great tuberosity				
Elbow 0			Capitellum			Head of radius
Hand 0	Hamate (4 *mths.*) Capitate (6 *mths.*) Ep. radius			Triquet-rum Ep. meta-carpals Ep. phalanges	Lunatum	Trapez-ium Scaphoid
Hip 0	Head of femur (9 *mths.*)				Great troch-anter	
Knee Ep. femur and tibia					Head of fibula	Patella
Foot Cuboid	Ext. cuneiform Ep. tibia	Ep. fibia		Int. cuneiform Ep. meta-tarsals	Mid cuneiform Navicular	

The new centres of ossification which appear at each year are shown in black. From Lawson Wilkins, *The Diagnosis and Treatment of Endocrine Disorders in Childhood and Adolescence* (3rd edit., 1965). Courtesy of Charles C. Thomas, Publisher, Springfield, Illinois.

CHRONOLOGICAL ORDER OF APPEARANCE OF UNION OF EPIPHYSIS WITH DIAPHYSIS

6	7	8	9	10	11 yrs.
Union head and tuberosity					
Int. epicondyle			Trochlea Olecranon		Ext. epicondyle
Trapezoid Ep. ulna				Pisiform	
	Union ischium & pubis			Ep. lesser trochanter	
					Tibial tubercle
		Ep. os calcis			

The new centres of ossification which appear at each year are shown in black. From Lawson Wilkins, *The Diagnosis and Treatment of Endocrine Disorders in Childhood and Adolescence* (3rd edit., 1965). Courtesy of Charles C. Thomas, Publisher, Springfield, Illinois.

RESPIRATORY FUNCTION TESTS

Normal values (with 95% confidence limits) for forced vital capacity (FVC), forced expiratory volume in one second ($FEV_{1.0}$) and peak expiratory flow rate (PEFR) in relation to height, in litres and corrected for body temperature and barometric pressure (LBTPS). L/S = litres/sec.

Height (cm)	FVC (LBTPS) (2 SD's ±26%)	$FEV_{1.0}$ (LBTPS) (2SD's ±18%)	PEFR (L/S) (2SD's ±26%)
110	1·21 (0·90–1·52)	1·09 (0·89–1·29)	150 (110–190)
120	1·53 (1·13–1·93)	1·39 (1·14–1·64)	200 (150–250)
130	1·90 (1·41–2·39)	1·74 (1·43–2·05)	255 (190–320)
140	2·32 (1·72–2·92)	2·14 (1·75–2·53)	310 (230–390)
150	2·79 (2·06–3·52)	2·60 (2·13–3·07)	360 (265–455)
160	3·32 (2·46–4·18)	3·12 (2·56–3·68)	410 (305–520)
170	3·91 (2·89–4·93)	3·69 (3·03–4·35)	455 (335–575)

From Polgar and Promadhat, *Pulmonary Function Testing in Children* (1971). Philadelphia: W. B. Saunders Company.

REFERENCES

DRILLIEN, C. M. and DRUMMOND, M. B. (1977). *Neurodevelopmental Problems in Early Childhood*. Oxford: Blackwell Scientific Publications.

HOLT, K. S. (1977). *Developmental Paediatrics: Perspective and Practice* (Postgraduate Paediatric Series). London: Butterworth.

ILLINGWORTH, R. S. (1980). *The Development of the Infant and Young Child: Abnormal and Normal*, 7th edit. Edinburgh: Churchill Livingstone.

SHERIDAN, MARY D. (1975). *The Developmental Progress of Infants and Young Children*, 3rd edit. London: H.M.S.O. (Min. of Health, No. 102).

II
NUTRITION

A guide to advisable intakes of nutrients is given in Table I.

Younger Infant (Birth till weaning)

Breast feeding.—Antenatal preparation is important in promotion of breast feeding. The baby receives colostrum which is rich in trace elements and anti-infective factors during the first two days of breast feeding after which mature milk "comes in". Thereafter the baby may wish to feed as often as two-hourly but more usually 3- or 4-hourly. Successful breast feeding ensures close contact between mother and child and minimises the risk of bacterial contamination of the milk. Breast milk itself has advantages over unmodified cow's milk in that the concentrations of protein, phosphorus and major minerals are lower, the fat is more easily absorbed, quality of the protein may be more suitable in the early days of life and it contains anti-infective substances, e.g. lactoferrin and maternal IgA. Vitamin supplements are often recommended for breast-fed infants (5 drops daily of the DHSS mixture—see p. 23).

Bottle feeding.—Feeding usually commences during first 8 hours of life and continues every 3–4 hours thereafter, eventually missing out the night feed to give *approximately* a 4-hourly, 5 times a day, regular, but flexible, routine. One of the formulae shown in Table II is recommended. It is fed to satisfy appetite which will be approximately 150 ml per kg per day (120–180 ml) during the first 4 months of life. This will supply all the necessary nutrients, but vitamin supplements may be recommended (see p. 23). Great care is needed in reconstitution of the feeds, e.g. cleaning and sterilising of bottles, teats, etc., measuring of fluid and scoops of powder, particularly to avoid too concentrated feeds, and handling of feed after reconstitution to avoid bacterial growth.

Older Infant (Weaning till first birthday)

Mixed feeding usually starts between 3 and 6 months. Too early introduction of mixed feeding may contribute to renal osmolar load problems, obesity in Britain, undernutrition in developing countries, and development of coeliac disease in the young infant. Too late introduction might (theoretically)

TABLE I

DAILY INTAKES IN HEALTHY CHILDREN

Age (years)	Younger[a] infant 0–5/12	Older infant 6–11/12	Toddler 1–4	Primary schoolchild 5–11	Secondary schoolchild 12–18
	Intake per kg body wt	Total intake per day			
Energy					
MJ	0·430	3·8–4·2	5–7	7–10	10–13
kcal	100	910–1000	12–1600	18–2400	25–3000
Protein (g)	1·5	23–25	30–40	45–60	60–75
Vitamins					
A (retinol μg)	90	150	300	300–600	750
Thiamine mg	0·03	0·2	0·6	0·7–1·0	1·0
Nicotinic acid mg	1	5	7–9	10–14	16–19
C mg	6	20	20	25	30
D (chole-calciferol μg)	5[b]	10	10	2·5	2·5
Sodium mmol	1·0	6[c]	8[c]	50[c]	100[c]
Potassium mmol	2·3	6	8	20	50
Magnesium mmol	0·2	1·0	1·0	10	15
Calcium mmol	1·3	9	13	13–18	18
Iron mmol	0·002	0·1	0·15	0·2	0·25
Water litres [d]	0·12–0·18	0·8–1·2	1–1·5	1–1·5	1·2–1·5

Notes: (a) Figures for younger infant are those contained in 150 ml of human milk.

(b) As vitamin D sulphate; specificity and anti-rachitic property doubtful.

(c) Electrolytes in older infants and toddlers mainly from Fomon (1974) *Infant Nutrition* (Philadelphia: W. B. Saunders). Much higher intakes are common, but are not necessary; in school children figures are based on observed intakes.

(d) This does not include water found in solid food; a fully mixed diet may contribute the same volume of water again; total water requirements are related to energy and solute content of diet.

Other figures mainly from DHSS (1979) *Recommended Intakes of Nutrients*.

Atomic weights: Sodium 23, Potassium 39, Magnesium 24, Calcium 40, Iron 56. Energy value of nutrients (kJ per g): protein 17, carbohydrate 16, fat 37. 1 MJ = 240 kcal. 1 kcal = 4·2 kJ.

lead to deficiency of trace elements and (if on unmodified cow's milk) essential fatty acids or refusal to chew and swallow solid food.

A teaspoonful of baby rice mixed with water or milk may be given before a milk feed and the amount gradually increased. Other foods (commercially available or home prepared) are then introduced, such as broth, mixed sieved vegetables, mashed potatoes and gravy, milk puddings, fish, minced meat, etc., and up to 600 ml of milk should be continued throughout infancy.

After introducing mixed feeding, breast feeding or one of the formulae shown in Table II may be continued, or doorstep milk may be substituted. If doorstep milk is used, vitamin supplements are essential (see below) and because of the high renal solute load of doorstep milk the infant will probably want extra water. In developing countries breast feeding should be encouraged for many months after introducing mixed feeding, well into the second year of life.

Vitamin supplements.—Five drops (0·15 ml) of the British DHSS vitamin drops contain vitamin A 214 μg as retinol (714 iu), vitamin C 21 mg and vitamin D 7 μg (calciferol 290 iu); the recommended dose is 5 drops daily.

This supplement should be given to *all* young children unless the medical attendant is sure that the child is receiving an adequate supply of vitamin D from the sun and other dietary sources.

It is usually not essential for the formula-fed baby or the breast-fed baby of a well-nourished mother, but it is essential for infants receiving doorstep milk and for most Asian children.

Certain special milks and formulae may need additional vitamin supplementation. See Table VI, pp. 34–35.

Toddlers (1–4-year-olds)

By his first birthday the British child is usually eating three or four meals a day, preferably with other members of the family and from the same menu. Many children will continue to drink up to 500 ml of doorstep milk during their toddler years and this provides a substantial proportion of their intake of protein (18 g), calcium (15 mmol) and riboflavine (700 μg). A few drink very little milk, however, with no obvious ill-health. Many mothers become worried by an apparently poor

TABLE II
ANALYSIS OF MILK FORMULAE (PER LITRE RECONSTITUTED FEED)

	Energy MJ (kcal)	Protein g	Fat g	Carbohydrate g	Vitamin A µg (a) retinol	Vitamin C mg	Vitamin D µg (b) calciferol	Sodium mmol	Potassium mmol	Magnesium mmol	Calcium mmol	Phosphorus mmol	Iron mmol
Suitable for younger and older infants													
Human milk	2·8 (690)	10	42	74	600	38	0·1	7	15	1·2	9	5	0·01
Cow and Gate Plus	2·7 (650)	19	35 (c)	69	800	53	11	12	22	—	17	17	0·1
Premium	2·8 (680)	15 (d)	38 (c)	72	800	53	11	8	15	1·8	10	10	0·1
Milumil	2·8 (690)	19	31 (c)	84	570	75	10	13	22	—	18	18	0·1
Ostermilk Complete	2·7 (650)	17	27	86 (e)	1050	64	10	13	21	2·5	14	15	0·2
SMA	2·7 (650)	15	35 (c)	70	800	53	11	11	19	2·3	13	14	0·2
Gold Cap SMA–S26	2·8 (670)	15 (d)	36 (c)	72	800	63	11	7	14	2·0	11	11	0·1
New Ostermilk Two	2·6 (630)	18	25	83 (f)	1050	63	10	13	21	2·5	14	15	0·1
New Osterfeed	2·8 (680)	15 (d)	38	70	1040	69	10	7	15	2·0	9	10	0·1
Doorstep cow's milk	2·8 (660)	33	37	48	400	16	0·6	25	36	5·0	31	31	0·02

Notes:
(a) 1 µg retinol = 3·3 iu vitamin A.
(b) 1 µg cholecalciferol = 40 units vitamin D.
(c) Contains vegetable and animal oils other than cow's milk fat.
(d) Modified cow's milk protein, curd : whey protein ratio similar to human milk.
(e) Approximately 30 g lactose, rest maltodextrins (hydrolysed starch).
(f) Approximately 53 g lactose, rest maltodextrins.

appetite, food fads, and a lack of variety in the foods accepted by the child at this age. Comparing the child's weight and height to growth charts usually shows that they are normal and nutritional analysis of many of these diets, which at first glance seem of limited value, often shows them to be quite adequate. Reassurance that the child will grow out of these food fads is often all that is required. However, some children who truly have a low energy consumption are lighter than average and a few who present with short stature in Britain at this age have a limited and capricious diet. They may require further investigation.

Obesity may develop at this age or during the school years and a few remain obese in adult life. Many children who were obese in late infancy are no longer so by the age of school entry.

In developing countries, however, mortality rates in toddlers are sometimes 30 times higher than in Britain due mainly to the combined effects of protein-energy malnutrition and infection.

SICK CHILDREN

Infancy

The regime described for mild gastro-enteritis (see p. 117) is also suitable for the feverish anorexic infant with, e.g., respiratory tract, or urinary tract infection. During this temporary period of higher fluid losses the aim is to give extra "free" water, reintroducing the normal diet gradually. Wherever possible breast feeding should continue during the illness to maintain lactation—particularly in developing countries.

Older Children

The aim is to maintain the advisable fluid intake (see Table I, p. 22) and to encourage the child to take an extra amount (2–5 per cent of body weight is a guide) if he is pyrexial, dyspnoeic or has loose stools. The choice of fluid is largely dictated by what the child will take. Mineral waters, tea, milk, etc., are all suitable, but the mineral waters and milk are preferably diluted with some water to reduce the sugar content. Ice lollipops, ice cream and jellies are a useful way of giving extra water. Solid foods are reintroduced after a few days as appetite returns.

FLUID DIET TO GIVE BY MOUTH, BY INTRAGASTRIC TUBE OR INTRAJEJUNAL TUBE

These diets are suitable for a child who has near normal gastro-intestinal, metabolic, cardiac and renal function, but who cannot take food normally, e.g. in coma, prolonged anorexia, abnormalities of nasopharynx and oesophagus.

Young Infant.—The formulae recommended for the young infant (see p. 24) may all be given by tube.

Older infant, toddler and schoolchild.—When tube feeding is required for a short period (10 days or less) a simple mixture shown in Table III may be used. For children over 5 years one of the liquid feeds in Table VII may be used. Their use in younger children is not fully established.

Tube Feeding Technique

To pass an *intragastric* tube, the distance from nose to xiphisternum is marked on the tube; the tube is moistened with water and then gently pushed into the nose of the child—pushing backwards rather than upwards—until the mark is reached. To confirm that the tube is in the stomach test aspirate with litmus paper. If in place secure the tube to the

TABLE III

FLUID DIET FORMULA

Ingredients		Nutritional value per litre of feed	
Doorstep milk	800 ml	Protein	26 g
Prosparol or Double Cream	50 ml	Fat	55 g
Sucrose or Caloreen	60 g	Carbohydrate	98 g
Tap water, make up to 1 litre		Energy	4·1 MJ
			(990 kcal)
		Sodium	20 mmol
		Magnesium	4 mmol
		Potassium	29 mmol
		Calcium	25 mmol

1. Give sufficient to meet energy requirements shown in Table I (p. 22) or as an alternative rule after the first birthday give 1200 ml of the mixture, plus an extra 100 ml for each year of age up to a maximum of 2½ litres, e.g. 3-year-old—1500 ml, 15-year-old—2500 ml.
2. Give Abidec 0·6 ml daily.
3. For longer term, note that this diet is high in calcium and deficient in iron.

child's cheek with adhesive tape. If the tube is of polyvinyl, or similar material, it may remain *in situ* for about a week. Feeds should be given about every 3 hours to young infants, more frequently to low birth weight babies, and less frequently to older children.

A *nasojejunal* tube is passed into the stomach as above and then allowed to pass by peristalsis into the duodenum or jejunum. Its position is first checked by aspirating fluid alkaline to litmus and then it should be confirmed by X-ray.

Sialastic tubes are preferable as they do not harden as do those made of PVC, but they are more difficult to introduce. Feeds should be given at least 2-hourly and preferably by continuous drip or pump.

COMMON PRIMARY NUTRITIONAL DISORDERS IN BRITAIN

Obesity

"Simple" obesity is usually associated with increased height and bone age—retardation in either suggests the obesity is part of some other syndrome. Treatment is difficult, amounting to dietary restriction only; prevention is therefore preferable.

Scurvy

This can occur in late infancy but is now very rare in Britain. The child may present with bleeding gums, fine purpura or a pseudo-paralysis due to subperiosteal haemorrhage.

Treatment: ascorbic acid orally 500 mg once, then 100 mg daily for one week, then prophylactic dose 25 mg daily.

Prevention: see Vitamin Supplements, page 38.

Rickets

In Britain, Asian infants and adolescents, and older infants receiving doorstep milk without vitamins, may develop rickets. Other causes of rickets, e.g. anticonvulsant therapy, malabsorption, renal glomerular and tubular disease and hypophosphatasia are much rarer causes, but must be considered particularly in a child not in one of the above groups.

Treatment in infancy: Vitamin D (calciferol) orally, 75 μg

(3000 units) daily until healing of bones has occurred and serum alkaline phosphatase is normal, then prophylactic dose 7 µg (300 units) daily. In developing countries where daily treatment may be difficult, a single I.M. dose of 1500 µg (60,000 units) calciferol may be given.

This regime will cure primary nutritional rickets and that due to malabsorption or anticonvulsants; it will not cover up instances of renal glomerular or tubular rickets.

Prevention: see Vitamin Supplements, page 38.

Iron-Deficiency Anaemia

Preterm babies, twins, older infants in whom weaning has been delayed, and toddlers who dislike meat or vegetables, often develop iron-deficiency anaemia. The possibility of blood loss, particularly from the gastro-intestinal tract should be considered; malabsorption may present this way, and sometimes apparent iron deficiency anaemia is really thalassaemia or lead poisoning.

Treatment: (*a*) An oral iron preparation is usually adequate in infancy, e.g. ferrous sulphate BP 60 mg (12 mg elemental iron) three times daily. Double these doses in toddlers.

(*b*) Parenteral iron is rarely necessary and is probably better avoided if the plasma transferrin concentration is low, e.g. in the newborn, the malnourished, or those with protein loss.

(*c*) Blood transfusion is occasionally necessary, e.g. if there is heart failure; frusemide should be given with the blood and 10 ml per kg of blood only should be infused over at least 6 hours (see p. 169).

(*d*) Source of blood loss (if any) should be treated; in some countries the most common cause is hookworm infestation (see p. 110).

Prevention: For preterm babies and twins 6–12 mg elemental iron daily throughout infancy. Oral prophylactic iron should not be given if the baby is breast feeding to avoid saturating the lactoferrin.

Most formulae contain 0·02 mmol (1 mg) of elemental iron per 100 ml which is sufficient for normal babies.

Other iron-containing foods, e.g. iron-fortified cereals, green vegetables, egg, should be introduced between the 3rd and 6th month of life.

COMMON PRIMARY NUTRITIONAL DISORDERS IN DEVELOPING COUNTRIES

Protein Energy Deficiency

Mild degrees of deficiency of energy and protein cause growth retardation; extreme degrees cause the syndromes of nutritional marasmus and kwashiorkor.

Treatment: Diet is the essential part of treatment but care is necessary with common complications such as hypothermia, hypoglycaemia, drowsiness, diarrhoea, heart failure, and infection. Using some of the foods shown in Table IV (p. 30) it is possible, using locally available products, to devise a diet which will provide 400–650 kJ (97–156 kcals), 2–4 g milk protein, 4–6 mmol potassium, 1–2 mmol magnesium and less than 3 mmol sodium per kg body weight each day. A selection of milk-based diets are shown in Table IV. During the second week of treatment solids are added to the milk diet.

Vitamin A Deficiency

Vitamin A deficiency is a major cause of blindness, particularly in the Middle East and South East Asia. Conjunctival keratosis and Bitot's spots occur, clouding of the cornea (xerosis) is a clinical emergency because it may go on to necrosis (keratomalacia) with scarring and sometimes perforation.

Treatment: Retinol (water miscible preparation) 3000 µg per kg body weight I.M. immediately.

3000 µg per kg body weight orally daily, days 2 to 6.

1500 µg daily thereafter until eyes are normal.

Associated kwashiorkor or marasmus should be treated at the same time.

Prophylaxis: Retinol (oily preparation) 300 µg daily by mouth, or 60,000 µg by mouth every 4 to 6 months (limited value only).

Infantile Beriberi

This condition occurs in South East Asia in breast-fed infants of thiamine-deficient mothers who eat a polished rice diet.

In the cardiac form a diuresis within a few hours of giving parenteral thiamine hydrochloride—25 mg I.V. or 100 mg I.M.—is diagnostic as well as therapeutic. This emergency

TABLE IV (a)
Casilan Dried Skimmed Milk-Sucrose Diet (CaDSu) for Children with Kwashiorkor

Ingredients of the "dry" CaDSu diet		Nutritional value per 100 ml reconstituted diet	
Casilan	33 g	Protein	4·0 g
Dried skimmed milk	30 g	Fat	6·1 g
Sucrose	30 g	Carbohydrate	4·6 g
Cottonseed oil	60 g	Energy	375 kJ
Potassium chloride	2·7 g	Potassium	4·7 mmol
Magnesium chloride	0·3 g	Magnesium	0·7 mmol
		Sodium	0·9 mmol
Total	156 g		

The mixture of "dry" ingredients is prepared for use by taking 156 g of this mixture and making it into a paste with a little cold boiled water in scalded equipment, and then adding, gradually, enough cold sterile water to make a total of 1000 g. The reconstituted diet is fed at the rate of 100 ml per kg of body weight per day. Add Abidec 0·6 ml and folic acid 1 mg daily.

TABLE IV (b)
Milk-Sucrose Diet (MSu) for Children with Marasmus

Ingredients of the "dry" mixture		Nutritional value per 200 g of the reconstituted diet	
Full-cream milk powder	80 g	Protein	4·0 g
		Fat	14·3 g
Sucrose	35 g	Carbohydrate	13·2 g
Cottonseed oil	50 g	Energy	840 kJ
		Potassium	5·2 mmol
		Magnesium	0·8 mmol
Total	165 g	Sodium	2·8 mmol

The mixture of "dry" ingredients is prepared for use by taking 165 g of this mixture and mixing as for CaDSu in Table IV (a).

The reconstituted diet is fed at the rate of 200 g per kg body weight per day or to capacity.

treatment is followed by 25 mg I.M. daily for three days, then 10 mg orally twice a day. The mother should be treated at the same time—10 mg orally twice a day. Treatment for other forms is the same.

Pellagra

Pellagra occurs in children usually of school age receiving a maize diet, particularly in South Africa. Evidence of general undernutrition is usually present, as well as the classical dermatitis on exposed areas.

Treatment should include nicotinamide orally 50 mg three times a day but a good mixed diet, including milk (to provide tryptophan) and supplements of the other B vitamins is necessary too. Very rarely intravenous nicotinamide 3 mg is necessary in the presence of severe anorexia and diarrhoea.

Prophylaxis: Diet should contain milk.

Iodine Deficiency

Goitres due to iodine deficiency may occur, particularly in adolescent girls, in many parts of the world; frank hypothyroidism is also occasionally present.

Treatment: Iodine 200 μg daily for 6 weeks, then 100 μg daily for prophylaxis.

DIETARY MANAGEMENT IN OTHER DISORDERS

Many transiently ill children require dietary attention and the diet may be an important aspect of the long-term treatment of many metabolic and gastro-intestinal disorders. This section gives details of diets in common use. A dietitian will be able to offer fuller and more varied regimes. *Diets for Sick Children* (1974), by D. E. M. Francis (Oxford: Blackwell Scientific), is useful for reference, and for proprietary preparations the manufacturer's data sheets should be consulted. For many of the disorders dietary manipulation is only one aspect of management.

SPECIAL FORMULAE AND DIETS

Tables V to VIII give details of special formulae, food supplements, individual nutrients, and thickening agents in common use.

Table IX and the following pages give details of foods and special diets suitable for the older infant, toddler and schoolchild. Considerable skill is necessary to design, for children of this age, a diet which is therapeutically suitable and still attractive and palatable.

If a child's diet is very unusual, e.g. it is based on special formulae and/or isolated nutrients, then consideration of the quantity and quality of the nutritional intake is essential, i.e. the sources of nutrients (fluid, energy, protein, carbohydrate, fat), major minerals (sodium, potassium, magnesium, calcium, iron), vitamins (including the less commonly considered ones, e.g. inositol, biotin) and trace elements. It is often necessary to supplement such diets with vitamin and/or mineral mixtures (see p. 38). For lists of special milks and formulae requiring such supplementation see page 34.

Many of the formulae and foods detailed in the Tables are prescribable (see section on "Borderline Substances" in a current *MIMS*). FP10 forms should be headed "as ACBS".

Key to Abbreviations Used

Nutrient Source:

(*a*) Protein	CM	Cow's milk (mainly casein)
	HC	Hydrolysed casein
	AA	Amino acids
	EAA	The eight essential acids for adults (i.e. no histidine or cysteine)
(*b*) Fat	BF	Butter fat from cow's milk
	V	Vegetable derived (high proportion of polyunsaturated long-chain)
	MCT	Medium chain triglyceride, saturated fat
(*c*) Carbohydrate	F	Fructose
	G	Glucose
	L	Lactose (glucose and galactose)
	S	Sucrose (glucose and fructose)
	HSt	Hydrolysate starch (glucose, maltose and higher dextrins). Sometimes referred to as maltodextrin or corn syrup solids
	St	Starch

TABLE V

SUMMARY OF NUTRITIONAL PROPERTIES OF SPECIAL FEEDS
(Greater detail is given in Table VI)

| Product | Protein | | Carbo-hydrate | Fat | | | | Others | | |
	Hydrolysed Casein or Non-Milk protein	Protein Content 15 g/l or less	Low Lactose/Galactose (traces only)	Sucrose/Fructose free	Low fat below 20 g/l	High proportion of Unsaturated Fats	Some fatty as Medium Chain Triglycerides	Energy Content below 2·5 MJ (600 kcals) per litre	Low Sodium below 11 mmol/l	Vitamin and/or Mineral supplements required (see Table VI)
Albumaid Hydrolysate Complete	+		+*	+	+*			+	+	+
Allergilac				+				+		+
Comminuted Chicken	+		+*	+	+			+	+	+
Edosol				+		+			+	+
Formula S	+		+	+		+				
Galactomin 17			+	+		+		+	+	+
Galactomin 18			+	+	+	+		+	+	+
Galactomin 19			+		+	+		+	+	+
Locasol				+		+				+
MCT (1) Milk			+			+	+**		+	+
Nenatal				+		+	+		+	
Nutramigen	+		+*			+				
Portagen			+*			+	+			
Pregestimil	+		+*			+	+			
Premium				+		+			+	
Prosobee (Liq)	+					+				
Prosobee (Pwd)	+		+			+			+	
SMA		+		+		+				
SMA Gold Cap		+		+		+			+	
Velactin	+		+			+			+	
Wysoy	+		+*			+			+	

* Completely Free
** Completely MCT Oil

Product		Allergilac (C & G)	Comminuted Chicken (C & G)	Edosol (C & G)	Formula S (C & G)	Galactomin 17 (C & G)	Galactomin 18 (C & G)	Galactomin 19 (C & G)	Locasol (C & G)	Lofenalac (M Jo)
Recommended Dilution w/v%		12½	50	12½	12½	12½	12½	12½	12½	15
Protein g Source		34 CM	38 chicken	35 CM	20 Soya & Methionine	28 CM	28 CM	28 CM	27 CM	23[1] HC
Fat g Source		20 BF	13–20 chicken	35 V	30 V	28 V	18 V	18 V	29 V	28 V
Carbohydrate g Source		54 L	nil	47 L	68 G HSt	63 HSt tr L	73 HSt tr L	73 F tr L	65 L	91 St HSt
Minerals mmol	Na	59	2·5	1·5	13	5·7	5·7	5·7	10·5	14·4
	K	35	6·4	22·5	16	14·6	14·6	14·6	19	18·3
	Ca	26	1·1	29·8	13·8	22·5	22·5	22·5	<1·6	16·5
	P	28	7·3	27	12·9	19·3	19·3	19·3	16·3	16
Vitamins to be given[2] Mineral mixture required[2]			special YES	special YES	special		special YES	special YES	special YES	special yes but *not* Ca	
Energy Value/L MJ (kcals)		2·2 (520)	1·3 (300)	2·6 (630)	2·5 (600)	2·1 (500)	2·3 (540)	2·3 (550)	2·5 (600)	2·9 (700)

[1] Deficient in phenylalanine.
[2] See Table VIII and note that in the expected lifetime of this book many of these feeds will be modified so that they no longer need supplements.

VI

FEEDS—PER LITRE OF
FEED

Minafen (C & G)	MCT (1) Milk (C & G)	Nenatal (R)	Nutramigen (M Jo)	Portagen (M Jo)	Pregestimil (M Jo)	Prosobee (Liq) (M Jo)	Prosobee (Pwd) (M Jo)	Velactin (W)	Wysoy (Wy)	Product
15	12½		15	15	15	50	15	15	13½	Recommended Dilution w/v%
25[1]	32 CM	18 CM	23 HC	25 CM	19 HC	20 Soya	20 Soya& Meth-ionine	18 Soya & Meth-ionine	21 Soya & Meth-ionine	Protein g Source
62 V	35 MCT	45 40% MCT 60% v	27 V	34·1 87% MCT 13% V	27 42% MCT 58% V	36 V	36 V	29 V	36 V	Fat g Source
96 G HSt	51 HSt tr L	74 68% GHst 32% L	89 S St	82·4 HSt. S	91 HSt	69·0 HSt	67 HSt	93 G.Hst 2% S	69 HSt.S	Carbohydrate g Source
28	5·4	8·7	14	14·6	13·7	12·6	10·9	5·2	8·7	
16	16·6	15·0	18	22·8	18·7	17·6	15·4	20·5	19	Minerals
35	30·8	25·0	16·1	16·7	15·7	15·8	15	15	15	mmol
12	26	16·0	15·6	16·2	13·6	16·2	12·9	20·9	14	
special	special YES									Vitamins to be given[2] Mineral mixture required[2]
4·2	2·6	3·2	2·9	2·9	2·8	2·8	2·8	2·8	2·8	Energy Value/L MJ
(1010)	(630)	(760)	(700)	(700)	(670)	(665)	(670)	(680)	(670)	(kcals)

TABLE VII

Composition of Dietary Supplements, Liquid Feeds, etc. per Kg of Food

Product, Manufacturer and recommended dilution (%) if any	Casilan (G)	Dried Skimmed Milk Powder (Domestic)	Forceval (Uni)	Aminutrin (Ge)	Albumaid Hydrolysate Complete (SHS)	Maxipro (SHS)	Maxijul (SHS)	Caloreen (R)	Calonutrin (Ge)	Hycal (Liquid) (B)	Sucrose (Table sugar)	Glucodin (G)	Liquigen (SHS)	MCT oil, M Jo, (Al, C & G, SHS)
	PROTEIN SUPPLEMENTS						CARBOHYDRATE SUPPLEMENTS						FAT SUPPLEMENTS	
Protein g	900	345	550	1000	894*	880	0	0	0	0	tr	0	0	0
Source	CM	CM	CM	AA	AA	CM								
Fat g	18	3	10	0	0	40	0	0	0	0	0	0	520	999
Source	BF	BF	BF			BF							MCT	MCT
Carbohydrate g	0	490	300	0	0	tr	1000	1000	1000	610	1000	1000	0	0
Source		L	L			L	HSt**	HSt*	HSt	HSt**	S	G		
Minerals mmol Na	4	260	<53	0	4	100	20	<18	40	6	0.2	—	17	0
K	tr	342	13	0	0.5	115	1	1	3	2	0.6	—	7	0
Ca	298	317	345	0	0.7	75	0	0	0	3	0.3	—	—	0
P	258	364	65	0	1	125	0	0	0	1.7	tr	—	—	0
Energy MJ (kcal)	16.2 (3860)	13.7 (3260)	15.4 (3670)	16.8 (4000)	15.0 (3576)	16.3 (3880)	16.8 (4000)	16.8 (4000)	16.8 (4000)	10.2 (2440)	16.8 (4000)	16.8 (4000)	16.8 (4000)	34.8 (8300)

* This value has been corrected for moisture content.

** Predominance of higher sugars resulting in a low osmolarity.

Category	Product, Manufacturer and recommended dilution (%) if any	Protein g	Protein Source	Fat g	Fat Source	Carbohydrate g	Carbohydrate Source	Na	K	Ca	P	Energy MJ (kcal)
FAT SUPPLEMENTS	Cream (Single) (Domestic)	24·0	CM	212	BF	32	L	18	32	19	14	9·2 (2190)
FAT SUPPLEMENTS	Cream (Double) (Domestic)	15·0	CM	482	BF	20	L	12	20	13	7	19·4 (4620)
FAT SUPPLEMENTS	Prosparol (DF)	0		500	V	0		0·7	0	0	0	18·9 (4500)
FAT SUPPLEMENTS	Corn Oil (Domestic)	tr		999	V	0		tr	tr	tr	tr	39·0 (9300)
POWDERS FOR LIQUID FEEDS	Build-up (C) 16%***	223	CM	5	BF	668	S & L	142	257	205	206	14·4 (3440)
POWDERS FOR LIQUID FEEDS	Complan (GI) 20%****	200	CM	160	V	546	LS & HSt	152	218	183	187	18·5 (4440)
LIQUID FEEDS	Clinifeed (R) 400***	40	CM	35·6		146	LS & HSt	27·9	33	10·6	19·7	4·5 (1064)
LIQUID FEEDS	Ensure (A)	37	CM (87% CM 13% soya)	36	V	145	S & HSt	32	33	13	17	4·3 (1030)
LIQUID FEEDS	Isocal (MJo)	34	CM	44	20% MCT 80% V	133	G HSt	23	34	15	17	4·3 (1030)
LIQUID FEEDS	Triosorbon (BDH) 30%	190	CM	190	80% MCT	560	HSt	200	200	60	90	19·8 (4705)
THICKENING AGENTS (Require cooking)	Arrowroot (Domestic) 2–4%	4		1		940	St	2	5	2	9	15 (3550)
THICKENING AGENTS (Require cooking)	Cornflour (Domestic) 2–4%	5		7		920	St	23	16	4	13	14·8 (3540)
THICKENING AGENTS (Require cooking)	Benger's (F) 4%	100	Wheat	12		830	St	130	36	4	35	16·0 (3800)
THICKENING AGENTS (Require cooking)	Sister Laura's 2–7%	144	Wheat	11		820	St					15·8 (3751)
THICKENING AGENTS	Carobel (C & G) 0·5–1%											
THICKENING AGENTS	Nestargel (N)											

Carobel (C & G) 0·5–1% and Nestargel (N): Nutrients not available for absorption

*** not chocolate flavour
**** plain vanilla or unflavoured

TABLE VIII

SOME AVAILABLE VITAMIN AND MINERAL SUPPLEMENTS (for indications see p. 34)

Preparation	Daily Recommended Dose	A µg	Thiamine	Riboflavin	Nicotinamide	Pyridoxine	C mg	D µg	Others	Sodium mmol	Potassium mmol	Magnesium mmol	Calcium mmol	Phosphorus mmol	Iron mmol	Trace elements
ADC Vitamin mixtures DHSS Vitamin drops	5 drops	214	—	—	—	—		7	—	—	—	—	—	—	—	—
ABIDEC* (Parke Davis)	0.6 ml (0.3 ml in infancy)	1200	1.0	0.4	5.0	0.5	21	10	—	—	—	—	—	—	—	—
Adexoline Liquid (Glaxo)	0.4 ml	420	—	—	—	—	42	14	—	—	—	—	—	—	—	—
Special Vitamin mixtures Cow & Gate (a) Vitamin Tablets	6 tablets at birth 8 tablets by i months onwards	—	3.0	3.0	10.0	1.0	120	—	E, K, B_{12} Pantothenate Folic Acid, Biotin	tr	—	—	—	—	0.2	Zn, Mn, Cu, Mb, I
Ketovite syrup	5 ml syrup	940	—	—	—	—	—	10	E, K, B_{12} Pantothenate Folic Acid Biotin, Choline, Inositol	—	—	—	—	—	—	—
plus Tablets (Paines & Byrne)	3 tablets	—	3.0	3.0	9.9	0.99	50	—		—	—	—	—	—	—	—
Aminogran (b) Mineral Mixture (A & H)	1.5 g/kg up to maximum of 8 g	—	—	—	—	—	—	—	—	1.7	2.1	0.4	2.1	1.9	0.01	Cu, Zn, Mn I, Al, Co, Mb
Metabolic (b) Mineral Mixture (SHS)	1.5 g/kg up to maximum of 8 g	—	—	—	—	—	—	—	—	1.7	2.1	0.4	2.1	1.9	0.01	Cu, Zn, Mn I, Al, Co, Mb

content per g of powder (for Aminogran and Metabolic Mineral Mixture rows)

(a) Contains sucrose; (b) if extra major minerals are not required, Cow & Gate tablets above may be suitable source of trace elements.

TABLE IX

Summary of Nutritional Properties of Special Foods for Older Children

Product	Gluten free	Lactose/ milk free	Sucrose/ fructose free	Low protein <0·5g%**	Low sodium <0·3 mmol %
Cow & Gate					
Glutenex Biscuits	+*	+			
Aminex Biscuits		+*	+*	+*	+*
Farmitalia Carlo Erba					
Aproten Pastas	+	+		+*	+
Aproten Crispbread	+	+		+*	+
Aproten Flour	+	+			+
Bi-Aglut Aproten Biscuits	+*				
GF Dietary Supplies					
Aglutella-Azeta Wafers	+*			+*	
Aglutella Pasta	+	+	+	+*	
dp chocolate cookies		+	+	+*	
GF Ener-G Rice Bran	+	+	+		
Ener-G Egg Replacer	+	+	+		
GF Brand Biscuits (Various)	+				
Juvela Gluten-free Mix	+*				
Juvela Protein-free Mix	+	+		+*	
Verkade Biscuits	+*				
Nistria (Low Sodium) Meat Products					+ (not all)
Glaxo-Farley					
Farley Rusk		+			+
Farley Baby Rice	+				
Gluten-free Biscuit	+*				
Rite-Diet					
Gluten-free Biscuits (various)	+*(not all)				
Gluten-free Breadmix	+*				
Gluten-free Baking Powder	+				
Gluten-free Tinned Bread (White or Brown)	+*	+		+*	
Gluten-free Flour	+*				
Low Protein and/or Low Sodium Tinned Bread	+	+	+	+*	+*
Low Protein Flour				+*	+
Low Sodium White Bread					+
Robinson					
Baby Rice	+	+	+	+	+

** Per average portion.   * Prescribable on FP10.
Manufacturers of foods for infants and toddlers provide up-to-date lists of their gluten-free, milk-free, dissacharide-free, etc., products.

Manufacturers

A	Abbott Laboratories Ltd., Queenborough, Kent
A & H	Allen and Hanburys Limited, London, E2 6LA
Al	Alembic Prods., Oaklands House, Oaklands Drive, Sale, Manchester M33
B	Beecham Prods. Ltd., Gt. West Road, Brentford, Middx.
BDH	BDH Pharmaceuticals Ltd., Lenten House, Lenten Street, Alton, Hants GU34 1JD
C	Carnation Foods Ltd., Bush House, Aldwych, London WC2B 4QA
C & G	Cow and Gate Baby Foods, Trowbridge, Wilts BA14 8HZ
D F	Duncan, Flockhart & Co. Ltd., Birkbeck Street, London E2
	Farmitalia Carlo Erba, Kingmaker House, Station Road, Barnet, Herts EN5 1NU
F	Fison Pharmaceuticals, 12 Derby Road, Loughborough, LE11 0BB
Ge	Geistlich Sons, Ltd., Newton Bank, Chester CH2 3QZ
	GF Dietary Supplies Ltd., Lowther Road, Stanmore, Middx HA7 1EL
Gl	Glaxo-Farley Foods Ltd., Plymouth, Devon PL3
M Jo	Mead Johnson, Stamford House, Langley, Slough, Berks SL3 6EB
N	Nestlé Co. Ltd., 36 Park Lane, Croydon, Surrey CR9 1NR
	Rite-Diet—Welfare Foods (Stockport) Ltd., London Rd. South, Poynton, Stockport SK12 1LA
R	Roussel Laboratories Ltd., Roussel House, Wembley Park, Middx HA9 0NF
S H S	Scientific Hospital Supplies, 38 Queensland Street, Liverpool L7 3JG
	Sister Laura's Infant Food, Springfield Works, Bishopbriggs, Glasgow
Uni	Unigreg Ltd., 15–17 Worple Road, London SW19
W	Wander Ltd., 42 Upper Grosvenor St., W1
Wy	Wyeth Laboratories, Huntercombe Lane South, Taplow, Maidenhead, Berks SL6 0PH

Gluten-free Diet for Coeliac Disease

In a gluten-free diet, all foods containing wheat and rye must be eliminated unless they have been specially treated to remove the gluten. It is best to avoid oats and barley too.

Foods allowed	**Foods forbidden**
Milk, cream, cheese, yoghurt.	Cheese spreads.
All meats and fish.	Sausages, meat and fish coated
Eggs, all fruits and vege-	with flour or breadcrumbs.
tables.	Tinned meat. Meat and fish
Butter, margarine vegetable	pasties.
oils, dripping, lard and cream.	Porridge. Breakfast cereals
Rice, tapioca, sago, cornflour	made from wheat or oats,
and custard powders.	e.g. Weetabix, Shredded
Breakfast cereals made from	Wheat, etc.
corn or rice, e.g. corn-	Semolina, spaghetti, mac-
flakes, Rice Krispies, gluten-	aroni and other pasta.
free bread, e.g. Rite-Diet.	Ordinary bread, cakes and
Sugar, honey, jam,	biscuits, flavoured crisps.
marmalade.	Malted bed-time drinks, e.g.
Tea, coffee, cocoa.	Horlicks.
Special products (see p. 39).	Certain chocolates, sweets
	and ice creams.

See p. 39 for details of gluten-free foods available on FP10. The Coeliac Society regularly publishes lists of gluten-free foods (P.O. Box 181, London NW2 2QY).

Minimal Galactose and Lactose Diet

Lactose is the disaccharide (glucose and galactose) found in milk and hence in all products made from or with milk. The minimal galactose diet shown is adequate for galactos-aemia, but occasionally even stricter limitation is necessary. Low-lactose diets are sometimes beneficial in gastro-intestinal disease and on occasion it may also be beneficial to limit the amount of sucrose, long-chain fat and gluten too. If special milk substitutes are used, a vitamin supplement may be required (see pp. 34, 35). An extended list of foods may be requested from a dietetic department.

Foods allowed	**Foods forbidden**
Prescribed Milk Substitute (see pp. 34, 35).	Milk, cream, butter, dried milk powders, cheese, yoghurt ice cream.
CoffeeMate* (for older children).	
Casilan.*	All tinned or prepared meats and fish or fish fingers.
Manufactured infant and toddler foods which *do not* include milk, milk solids, whey, cheese, lactose or monosodium glutamate. Check with manufacturers lists and labels carefully.	Sausages.
	Milk and fancy breads.
	All baby cereals with milk solids, e.g. Farex.
	Coco Krispies, Special K, Alpen-type cereals.
Freshly cooked plain meats and fish.	All other margarines.
Eggs.	All tinned milk puddings and tinned spaghetti with cheese.
All fresh vegetables and fruit.	Fudge, toffee, chocolate, crisps.
Baked beans except with sausage.	Complan, Carnation Instant Breakfast Food.
All bread, except milk and fancy breads. Farley's Rusks, Robinson's Baby Rice, Cow & Gate (Liga) Glutenex Rusk, Cornflakes, Rice Krispies Weetabix. Tomor margarine.	*All* drinking chocolate and malted milk powders.
	A large variety of manufactured foods contain skimmed milk and are unsuitable—check manufacturers' lists.
Outline spread, vegetable oils. Dry cereals and pastas cooked in water or with milk substitute. Jelly, boiled sweets, ice lollies (without ice cream/toffee centres), pastilles, gums, jam, syrup, sugar.	
Squash, fizzy pop, Oxo, Marmite and Bovril.	
Tea and coffee.	

* Contains milk-protein.

Low-sodium and Low-protein/High-protein Diets

These diets may be necessary in renal or liver disease. Sometimes potassium restriction is necessary too.

In Infancy

By choosing suitable formulae and supplements from Tables II, VI and VII it is possible to meet a variety of intakes.

Breast milk, Gold Cap SMA, Premium and Osterfeed are all in effect lower protein, lower sodium feeds. Diets which lead to an intake of protein or sodium below these levels should be used only with caution. The protein content of an individual feed may be increased without increasing its sodium content, by adding Casilan, but generally it is unwise for the protein to exceed 7 g per 100 ml of feed, or 10 g per 100 kcal of feed, or 10 g per kg body weight per day. At weaning, baby rice and/or special biscuits (see Table IX) may be introduced to children on a low-protein diet.

Older Child

Food supplements from Table VII (p. 37) may be useful additions to the child's self-selected meagre diet particularly for short-term use and when dietetic advice is not immediately available, e.g. "High-energy, low-protein, sodium, potassium": Caloreen, Hycal, Prosparol, etc. "High-protein, low-sodium": Casilan, Forceval, Aminonutrin, Maxipro, etc. Note that doorstep milk and skimmed milk contain large amounts of sodium and potassium relative to their protein and energy content.

For longer-term management food tables and exchange lists must be consulted; a dietitian's help is invaluable. If possible energy intake should be maintained at 10 per cent over the normal intake for age, and protein intake should rarely be less than half the normal (see Table I). The children are often anorexic and food supplements are necessary to maintain growth. Liquid food supplements may be more acceptable to the anorexic child as a "medicine" morning and evening. This allows him a more free diet during the day (in effect restricted by his anorexia).

Low-Fat Diet (approximately 25 g)

This diet may be of value in malabsorption. When limiting dietary fat care is necessary to avoid also limiting associated nutrients, e.g. energy, protein, and fat-soluble vitamins. In malabsorption medium-chain triglyceride (MCT) oil or formula introduced slowly and/or carbohydrate supplements (see Tables V and VI) if they are tolerated, may be used as an energy supplement.

Diets used for the treatment of the hyperlipidaemias are commonly more restricted in long-chain fat than the one shown below; depending on the variety of the hyperlipidaemia, extra energy may be provided by polyunsaturated oils or MCT oil.

Foods allowed	**Foods forbidden**
Skimmed milk liquid or powder, Casilan.	Ordinary doorstep milk, cream, butter, margarine, cheese, ice cream.
White fish, lean meat either boiled, grilled or roast with no additional fat.	Eggs. All oils. All fatty meats (bacon, ham).
All fruit and vegetables. Clear vegetable soups.	Oily fish, canned meat and fish.
Robinson's Baby Rice. All adult breakfast cereals. Dried cereals and pasta cooked with water or milk substitute. Meringues. Bread.	Pastry, pies, sausages, gravy. All fried foods. Chips, fried vegetables. Cream soups. All cakes and biscuits. Doughnuts, fancy buns.
Jelly, water/plain ice lollies. Jam, honey, syrup, sugar, boiled sweets, sugar.	Chocolate, toffee, crisps, nuts, fudge. Lemon curd, peanut butter.
Fruit juice and squashes, fizzy pop, Bovril, Marmite, Oxo. Tea and coffee.	All chocolate and malted milk powders.

Additional portions of fat would be provided by:

1 egg (7 g), 5 g margarine or butter (4 g), 10 g Outline margarine (4 g).

B.A.W.
A.deL.

[NOTES]

[NOTES]

[NOTES]

[NOTES]

[NOTES]

[NOTES]

III
FLUID AND ELECTROLYTE THERAPY
AND
PARENTERAL NUTRITION

FLUID AND ELECTROLYTE THERAPY

Fluid and electrolyte therapy involves three basic considerations:
1. Provision of maintenance requirements.
2. Replacement of pre-existing deficits.
3. Correction of continuing losses.

CALCULATION OF MAINTENANCE REQUIREMENTS

Maintenance requirements of fluid and electrolytes are proportional to the child's calorie needs. Sick children may require more or less than usual, depending upon their metabolic rates.

MAINTENANCE I.V. FLUID AND ELECTROLYTE REQUIREMENTS

Body Weight	Kilocalories*/day	Fluid ml/day	Sodium mmol/day	Potassium mmol/day
Less than 10 kg	100/kg	100–120/kg	2·5–3·5/kg	2·5–3·5/kg
10–20 kg	75–100/kg	90–120/kg	2·0–2·5/kg	2·0–2·5/kg
over 20 kg	45–75/kg	50–90/kg	1·5–2·0/kg	1·5–2·0/kg

* 1 kcal = 4·2kJ (kilojoules)

Maintenance fluid and sodium requirements are most conveniently administered as 0·18 per cent sodium chloride and dextrose 4 per cent. The glucose supplied does not satisfy calorie needs but will prevent the development of ketosis if oral feeding has been stopped. *Note that intravenous fluid requirements are less than oral.*

CALCULATION OF PRE-EXISTING DEFICIT

In practice, deficits are most easily expressed in terms of body weight, e.g. 5 per cent dehydration in 5 kg baby = 250 ml.
Estimation of Dehydration—expressed as a percentage of body weight.
mild—5%: decreased skin turgor;
dry mucous membranes.

moderate—10%: increased severity of above signs;
                 sunken fontanelle;
                 reduced intra-ocular pressure;
                 tachycardia, oliguria.
severe—15%: marked increase in severity of
                 above signs; shock,
                 drowsiness, hypotension.

Types of dehydration.—Three types are recognised, resulting from variable loss of sodium in relation to water:

    hypotonic – serum sodium < 130 mmol/l
    isotonic – serum sodium 130–150 mmol/l
    hypertonic – serum sodium > 150 mmol/l

The degree of dehydration may be underestimated in hypertonic states, due to increased tissue turgor.

PRACTICAL MANAGEMENT OF DEHYDRATION

Hypotonic and isotonic

1. *If the patient is more than 5 per cent dehydrated or is shocked.*
   Give an isotonic solution, such as 0·9 per cent saline, or plasma at 20 ml/kg I.V. over 1–2 hrs, then continue as 2. Monitor B.P. and urine output.
2. *If the patient is less than 5 per cent dehydrated and cannot tolerate oral fluids.*
   Replace the dehydration deficit as calculated as 0·18 per cent saline, or 0·45 per cent saline with dextrose if the serum sodium is 130 mmol/l or less, changing to 0·18 per cent saline in 4 per cent dextrose as the serum electrolytes improve. Add potassium chloride (3 mmol/kg/24 hrs) after urine flow is established and the blood urea is falling towards normal.
   A guide to the volumes needed is found on the next page.
3. Monitor serum electrolytes, and possibly H^+ concentration on admission and after 2, 12, and 24 hours. Record fluid intake and output accurately, and weigh the patient daily.
   I.V. fluids given to infants should always be administered

from a graduated chamber to prevent inadvertent sudden fluid overload.

Hypertonic (hypernatraemic) dehydration

Intracellular fluid loss predominates initially so that the classical features of dehydration and circulatory failure

ROUGH GUIDE TO REHYDRATION

(First 24 hours, excluding newborn)
Basic fluid will be 0·18 per cent saline in 4 per cent dextrose.

HYPOTONIC OR ISOTONIC DEHYDRATION Na<150 mmol/l		HYPERTONIC DEHYDRATION Na>150 mmol/l	
1. IF shocked or > 5% dehydration give initial infusion 20 ml/kg in 1–2 hours of 0·9% saline or plasma. Continue as in 2.		1. Give 20 ml/kg 0·9% saline or plasma in 1–2 hours	
2. Unless initial infusion required, START with 0·18% saline 4% dextrose at 150 ml/kg/day		2. Continue with 0·18% saline 4% dextrose at 100 ml/kg/day	
Wt (kg)	*ml/24 hr*	*ml/hr*	*ml/24 hr*	*ml/hr*
2	300	12	200	9
3	450	19	300	13
4	600	25	400	18
5	750	31	500	23
6	950	40	600	27
7	1050	44	700	32
8	1200	50	800	36
9	1350	56	900	41
10	1500	63	1000	45

For additions of bicarbonate or potassium and adjustment of sodium intake, see text.

develop slowly. The skin is of a doughy consistency and
neurological features may be prominent. Most cases result
from loss of hypotonic fluid, i.e. greater water than electrolyte
loss; however some may result from excess sodium administration. After circulating blood volume has been restored,
lower serum sodium slowly over 2–3 days to avoid CNS
disturbance. Hypocalcaemia may be present and should be
corrected.

Management

(1) Rehydration: Despite misleading appearances many
    infants require initial repletion of the circulating blood
    volume using plasma or 0·9 per cent saline, 20 ml/kg over
    1–2 hours. Thereafter maintenance solutions should be
    hypotonic, preferably 0·18 per cent saline in 4 per cent
    dextrose at a rate no faster than 100 ml/kg/24 hour.
(2) Urine collection: measure output, examine for deposit; if
    oliguria estimate urinary urea and electrolytes.
(3) If shocked record B.P. Normal values should be consis-
    tently obtained following initial infusion.

Delay correction of metabolic acidosis until initial rehydration is complete.

Potassium supplements are added as detailed under
"Hypotonic and isotonic dehydration". If oliguria persists and
hypernatraemia has resulted from excess sodium chloride
administration, peritoneal dialysis may be required.

Potassium Therapy

Plasma concentration is a poor guide to the total body
potassium, particularly in the presence of dehydration and
acidosis, in both of which it is raised. Potassium should be
given orally if possible and not commenced until urine flow is
established and the blood urea is falling. If given intravenously
add 3 mmol/kg/24 hr not exceeding a maximum concentration of 40 mmol/l. ECG monitoring is useful in difficult cases.
As intravenous therapy is being discontinued an oral rehydration preparation, e.g. Dioralyte, should be chosen which also
contains potassium, to continue to repair the total body
deficit. The management of hyperkalaemia is detailed in
Chapter VI, page 134.

Metabolic Acidosis

Metabolic acidosis will tend to correct spontaneously as the circulation and renal function improve and the electrolyte loss subsides. Estimation of the bicarbonate needed to correct acidosis is not precise. Over-rapid and full correction may increase CSF acidosis and produce apnoea. Theoretically, the amount of bicarbonate required is described by the formula:

base deficit $(mmol/l) \times$ body weight $(kg) \times 0.3 = mmol$ for full correction.

Not more than half this amount should be given over 24 hours. In the face of severe progressive acidosis (base deficit greater than 10 mmol/l), imminent collapse or situations where acidosis is unlikely to disappear with other I.V. fluids, an initial 0.5 mmol/kg may be given rapidly over 10 minutes and further 0.5 mmol/kg over the next hour. The remainder is then given over 24 hours if indicated by Astrup analysis.

Metabolic Alkalosis

This may occur following persistent vomiting as in pyloric stenosis, in cases of potassium loss and sodium retention, and following the administration of excess alkali. It is usually a self-correcting condition if renal function is good and the precipitating cause eliminated. If alkalosis is severe and tetany is imminent, it may be necessary to give ammonium chloride. The amount used is:

mmol chloride = base excess $(mmol/l) \times 0.3 \times$ body wt (kg)

[Inj. ammomium chloride is 0.89 per cent (1/6 molar) containing 167 mmol of each ion per litre.]

During a period of alkalosis excess potassium is lost in the urine. Extreme degrees of non-respiratory alkalosis may prove resistant to therapy until any potassium deficit is corrected.

Blood Volume

The infant's blood volume is 8 per cent (80ml/kg) of the body weight, so that a transfusion of 20 ml/kg whole blood will raise the haemoglobin by approximately 25 per cent.

CORRECTION OF CONTINUING LOSSES

These losses are usually from the gastro-intestinal or renal tract. Replacement should be contemporaneous, the fluids being of similar composition to those lost, their volume being calculated every 6–8 hours. In small infants with large continuing losses, waiting for a 24-hr period to calculate replacement is too long. Fortunately diarrhoea usually stops when the intravenous infusion has started and the replacement fluids calculated (at 5 per cent, etc) are generous. Mild ongoing diarrhoea is usually ignored and in practice its likely sodium content corresponds approximately to 0·18 per cent saline.

Electrolyte composition of alimentary fluids (mmol/l)

	H^+	Na^+	K^+	Cl^-	HCO_3^-
Gastric	40–60	20–80	5–20	100–150	—
Small Bowel	—	100–140	5–15	90–130	20–40
Biliary	—	120–140	5–15	80–120	30–50
Diarrhoea	—	40	40	40	40

In sodium depletion due to renal loss the urinary sodium concentration is high (> 40 mmol/l); when unrelated to renal disease urinary sodium concentration is extremely low (< 10 mmol/l).

COMPOSITION OF SOLUTIONS FOR INTRAVENOUS USE IN MMOL/L

	Na^+	K^+	Cl^-
Sodium chloride injection (0·9%)	150	—	150
Sodium chloride (0·18%) and dextrose (4%) injection	30	—	30
Hartmann's	130	4	104
Citrated plasma	150	12	55

1 ml of 8·4% sodium bicarbonate contains

1 mmol bicarbonate;
1 mmol sodium

1 ml Strong potassium chloride BP contains

2 mmol of potassium
2 mmol of chloride

1 ml 30 per cent sodium chloride contains

5 mmol of sodium
5 mmol of chloride

1 ml Inj. calcium gluconate B.P. 10% contains

0·225 mmol Ca^{++}

Calculation of millimoles

One millimole = molecular weight in milligrams.
Useful atomic weights:

hydrogen	1·0	magnesium	24·3
carbon	12·0	phosphorus	31·0
nitrogen	14·0	chlorine	35·5
oxygen	16·0	potassium	39·1
sodium	23·0	calcium	40·1

For example:
1 mmol NaCl = 58·5 mg. 1 mmol NaHCO$_3$ = 84 mg.
1 mmol KCl = 74·6 mg. 1 mmol NH$_4$Cl = 53·5 mg.

M.P-B.

PARENTERAL NUTRITION

Parenteral nutrition (PN) is achieved by the intravenous administration of amino acids, carbohydrates, fat, macro and micro elements, and vitamins. (It may be total or partial.)

Indications

1. When enteral feeding is inadequate to promote healing and leads to serious delays in recovery, particularly after gut surgery, trauma or burns.
2. When nutritional intake is so inadequate that normal brain growth may be imperilled, e.g. sick, low-birth-weight babies.
3. When the gut must be "rested" as in protracted diarrhoea unresponsive to other treatment, severe necrotising entero-colitis and some cases of inflammatory bowel disease.
4. After massive gut resection.
5. Prolonged paralytic ileus.

Techniques

PN may be given via either a central or peripheral vein and in some instances an artery or arteriovenous fistula. Catheters should be inserted using a strict aseptic technique and such catheters should only be used for PN and not for blood sampling.*

Composition of Fluid

Bags of fluid containing amino acids, glucose, macro and micro elements and vitamins should be made up by a pharmacist in a laminar flow unit. The volume of fluid required, nutrient content and the amounts of micro and macro elements and vitamins can be ascertained from Tables X and XI.

Patients should be fed initially for their actual weight and then when gaining weight by increments for their expected weight. Abnormal losses should be taken into account. Intralipid*† is dispensed separately. The volumes given refer to volume of fluid rather than water alone.

The equivalent of these fluid and nutrient allowances is shown in Table XII for commercially available fluids.

* Intralipid given over 20 hours per day; wait until infusion stopped four hours before taking blood samples.
† KabiVitrum.

TABLE X

INTRAVENOUS FLUID IN THE NEWBORN

Requirements according to age in days and birth weight.

Day of life	Volume (ml/kg)
1	60
2	75
3	90
4, 5	120
6	150
6+	150–200

add 30 ml/kg/day of water if naked baby under radiant heater or phototherapy lights.

The constituents and volume of the fluids should be adjusted for patients with heart, renal and liver disease or failure, as well as those with metabolic and nutritional abnormalities.

Amino acids.—This regime uses Vamin† 10 per cent glucose which is a crystalline L-amino acid solution with a profile similar to that of egg protein and one of the most suitable of those available for use in children. The amount should be reduced if the plasma urea and ammonia become elevated.

Carbohydrate.—Only glucose should be used. The amount infused should be reduced if glycosuria$>\frac{1}{2}$ per cent or blood sugar$>9\cdot7$ mmol/l (175 mg%) occurs. It is usually not necessary to use insulin if the glucose is introduced slowly. The concentration of glucose in the solution may be increased if the volume of infusate needs to be decreased without decreasing the calories.

Fat.—This should be given as 10 per cent Intralipid. This is an isotonic fat emulsion prepared from fractionated soybean oil with egg phosphatides. The fat is 85 per cent unsaturated and polyunsaturated triglycerides. Small-for-dates and preterm babies are liable to have a reduced plasma clearance. It should not be given if the plasma bilirubin>100 μmol/l, unless the bilirubin-binding capacity of the plasma can be measured. Neither should Intralipid be given when the patient has an uncontrolled infection. Energy derived from fat should not normally exceed 40 per cent of the total energy.

† KabiVitrum.

TABLE XI

PARENTERAL NUTRITION

Total requirements of nutrients and electrolytes per kg body weight calculated according to age or weight of infant or child and by day from start of parenteral nutrition.

	Day of Parenteral Nutrition	Fluid Volume (ml/kg)	Non N_2 (kcal/kg)	Amino acids (g/kg)	N_2 (g/kg)	Glucose (g/kg)	Fat (g/kg)	Sodium (mmol/kg)	Potassium (mmol/kg)
Requirements in newborn	Day 1	See Table X	42	0·5	0·07	8	1	3	2·5
	2		50	0·75	0·10	10	1	3	2·5
	3		60	1·0	0·13	10	2	3	2·5
	4		68	1·5	0·20	12	2	3	2·5
	5		86	2·0	0·27	14	3	3	2·5
	6		91–99	2·5	0·34	14–16	3·5	3	2·5
Requirements for babies > 1 month of age and < 10 kg	Day 1	150	42	0·5	0·07	8	1	3	2·5
	2	150	50	1·0	0·13	10	1	3	2·5
	3	150	68	1·5	0·20	12	2	3	2·5
	4	150	72	2·0	0·27	13	2	3	2·5
	5 and over	170	86	2·5	0·34	14	3	3	2·5
10–30 kg	Day 1 and 2	60–100	33	1·0	0·13	4·5	1·5	2–3	2–3
	3 and over	60–100	48–62	2·0	0·27	7–8	2–3	2–3	2–3
30 kg+	Day 1 and 2	40–75	18	1	0·13	2	1	2–3	2–3
	3 and over	40–75	32–62	1·5	0·20	3–8++	2–3	2–3	2–3

(a) Vitamins as in text.
(b) Macro and micro elements:
If weight < 10 kg add Ped-el 4 ml/kg/day
> 10 kg add Addamel 0·2 ml/kg/day
after checking text (p. 64).
++ increase glucose by 1 g/kg body wt/day if tolerated.

TABLE XII

SCHEME FOR PARENTERAL NUTRITION

(using commercially available products) All values are given per kg body weight per day

	Day of Parenteral Nutrition	Post-gestational age (days)	Fluid volume (ml)	Vamin** (ml)	5% dextrose (ml)	10% dextrose (ml)	10% Intralipid (ml)	Additional	
								Na (mmol)	K (mmol)
NEONATES INCLUDING LOW BIRTH WEIGHT According to day of age and length of parenteral nutrition in days	1	3	90*	7	—	73	10	2·7	2·4
	1	4 & 5	120*	7	60	43	10	2·7	2·4
	1	6 and over	150*	7	120	13	10	2·7	2·4
	2	4 & 5	120*	10	20	80	10	2·5	2·3
	2	6 and over	150*	10	80	50	10	2·5	2·3
	3	5	120*	14	60	86	20	2·3	2·2
	3	6 and over	150*	14	20	56	20	2·3	2·2
	4	6 and over	150*	21	—	89	20	2·3	2·1
	5	over 6	150–180*	28	—	112	30	1·6	1·9
	6	over 6	150–200*	35	—	105–125	35	1·25	1·8
INFANTS >1 month <10 kg	1		150	7	120	13	10	2·7	2·4
	2		150	14	80	46	10	2·3	2·2
	3		150	21	20	89	20	2·0	2·1
	4		150	28	—	102	20	1·6	1·9
	5 and over		170	35	—	105	30	1·25	1·8
10–30 kg	1 and 2		60	14	—	31	15	2·0	2·0
	3 and over		90–100	28	—	42–52	20–30	1·5	1·5
>30 kg	1 and 2		36	14	12	9–59***	10	2·0	2·0
	3 and over		50–75	21	—	9–59***	20–25	1·5	1·5

* If under radiant heater or receiving phototherapy allow 30 ml/kg/day of extra water. This may be achieved in most instances by reducing the 10 per cent dextrose by 30 ml/kg and increasing 5 per cent dextrose by 60 ml/kg.

** Vamin with 10 per cent glucose.

*** Volume of fluid may be decreased by substituting 20 per cent for 10 per cent dextrose.

(a) Vitamins as in text.
(b) Macro and micro elements:
If weight less than 10 kg add Ped-el 4 ml/kg/day.
When weight more than 10 kg add Addamel 0·2 ml/kg/day after checking text, page 64.

If Intralipid is not used, the infant's skin should be coated with sunflower oil twice daily to prevent essential fatty acid deficiency.

Macro and micro elements.—Vamin contains insufficient amounts of Na^+, K^+, Ca^{++}, Mg^{++}, and Cl^-. Sodium and potassium should be given as indicated in the Tables and increased to compensate for abnormal losses. Ped-el† contains Ca^{++}, Mg^{++}, Fe^{++}, Zn^{++}, Mn^{++}, Cu^{++}, F^-, I^-, P^{3-}, and Cl^- and is given to infants of up to 10 kg body weight in a dose of 4 ml/kg/day. It is added to the Vamin-dextrose solution when renal function has become established. There is no suitable electrolyte mixture commercially available for children over 10 kg, but Addamel† 0·2 ml/kg/day may be added to the Vamin-dextrose; it does not contain phosphate and has insufficient calcium. Trace element mixtures should only be given when renal function is established. Deficiencies particularly of zinc and copper are liable to occur in diarrhoeal states.

Vitamins.—Water-soluble vitamins should be given as Solivito†. The vial should be reconstituted with 5 ml of 10 per cent dextrose and added to the Vamin-dextrose or Intralipid in a dose of 0·5 ml/kg/day to a maximum of 5 ml/day. The solution must be protected from the light. Vitamins A, D and K can be given in the form of Vitlipid† 1 ml/kg/day to a maximum of 4 ml/day and must be added to the Intralipid.

Infusion System

This is shown diagrammatically in Fig. 1. Stringent asepsis is essential. Connections between the catheter and the infusion system should be soaked in isopropyl alcohol for 3 minutes before disconnection and reconnection of the fresh system. Millipore filters should be inserted on any air inlets. Fluid should not be allowed to enter the air inlet tubing. An air eliminator/particle filter should be included in the circuit as shown.

Nutrient solutions and the system should be changed daily and samples taken for bacteriology as indicated in Table XIII.

Monitoring

Table XIII gives the daily and weekly routines for monitoring of neonates, infants and children. The blood investigations

† KabiVitrum.

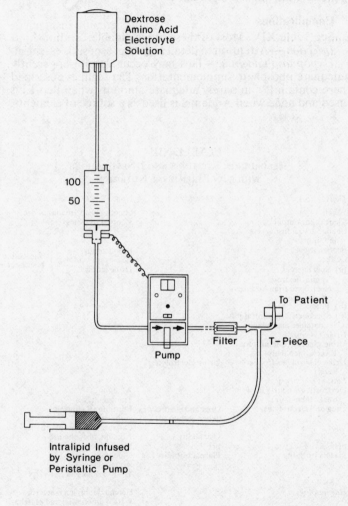

Fig. 1 – Diagram of infusion system used to administer parenteral nutrition.

should be performed with discretion as it is easy to exsanguinate a low-birth-weight baby.

Complications

See Table XIV. Most of these are avoidable.

Infection.—Attention to detail and strict asepsis is essential.

Hypophosphataemia.—This may occur despite apparently adequate phosphate supplementation. The regimes described here contain P^{3-} in barely adequate amounts when Ped-El is used and none when Addamel is used as a source of elements.

TABLE XIII
RECORDINGS, ROUTINES AND INVESTIGATIONS WHILE ON PARENTERAL NUTRITION

Daily	*3 ×Weekly*	*Once Weekly (or as indicated)*
Weigh		Length+head circumference
Chart input/output		Skinfold thickness
Change I.V. infusion sets and filters		
Bacteriology		
Culture		Blood culture ⎫ if infection
(a) Specimen of Vamin/dextrose electrolyte from burette or container.		CSF exam+culture ⎬ is suspected
(b) Filter		Urine culture ⎭
(c) Specimens from Intralipid container and tubing		
Urine Chemistry		
Urine glucose (6-hourly for 1 week, then daily)		
Urine electrolytes (for 1st week)	Urine electrolytes	
Plasma Chemistry		
Dextrostix (6-hourly for 1 week, then daily)		Albumin
		Transaminases
Urea and electrolytes	Urea and electrolytes (when stabilised)	Bilirubin (if clinically jaundiced)
		Calcium and phosphorus
	Osmolality	Alkaline phosphatase
pH	pH	Magnesium
Plasma turbidity	Plasma turbidity	Glucose
		Ammonia
		Triglycerides and free fatty acids
Haematology		Haemoglobin, haematocrit, WBC+differential and platelets
		Screening for blood coagulation defect (if indicated).

TABLE XIV

COMPLICATIONS OF PARENTERAL NUTRITION IN CHILDHOOD

Infection
Activation of infection
Electrolyte disturbances
Hypophosphataemia
    Anaemia
    Hypoxia
    Thrombocyte and neutrophil dysfunction
Hypo and hyperglycaemia
Trace element deficiencies
Hyperammonaemia
Hyper and hypocalcaemia
Essential fatty acid deficiency
Hepatic dysfunction
Increased folic acid requirement
Metabolic acidosis.

Phosphate is present as phospholipid in Intralipid although there is some suggestion that it may not be biologically available. If plasma levels fall below normal, phosphate should be given in a dose of 0·25–0·5 mmol/kg/day as the potassium salt in the daily requirement of dextrose solution. This cannot be mixed with Vamin or the trace element mixtures.

Hypoglycaemia.—To avoid this problem parenteral nutrition should never be stopped abruptly. Drips should be resited immediately and cessation of parenteral nutrition should be a gradual one as enteral feeding is increased.

Commencing Enteral Nutrition

This should be commenced cautiously and increased in volume and nutrient content depending on gastro-intestinal function. The parenteral nutrition should be reduced accordingly.

C.A.H.

[NOTES]

[NOTES]

[NOTES]

[NOTES]

[NOTES]

[NOTES]

[NOTES]

IV
THE NEWBORN

THE NEWBORN

The following points may give a clue to the nature of the baby's problems: maternal age, the medical and obstetric history, blood groups, antibodies, Wassermann reaction. The importance of an accurate record of the birth weight, gestation, cause of death and illness of siblings cannot be overstressed. A history of paternal disease, occupation and age can be relevant. In the current pregnancy record date of onset of last menstrual period (LMP) and expected date of delivery (EDD), complications and drugs, time of onset of labour, time of rupture of membranes and whether labour was spontaneous or induced. List drugs used in labour, the mode of delivery and calculate the membrane rupture/delivery interval. Note condition of the baby at birth, the Apgar scores, the time taken to breathe and nature of resuscitation required.

EXAMINATION OF THE BABY

Initial.—The baby should be briefly examined and assessed at birth. Oesophageal atresia should be excluded if there has been hydramnios. The aim is to assess the infant's general condition and his respiratory function and to determine whether any special management is required in the first few days. Generalised disorders such as Down's syndrome should be sought for at this time and imperforate anus, sexual ambiguity and single umbilical artery excluded. The examination, including a search for cleft palate, cataract, spinal or sacral dimple and dislocation of the hips should be completed and recorded within 24 hours.

On discharge, e.g. at 5–7 days, check that the baby is feeding well (and is gaining weight by seven days). If this is not the case, infection may have to be excluded and further observation and review arranged. Check that there is no superficial infection of skin, nails, eyes, mouth and umbilicus; listen to the heart; palpate femoral pulses and note presence and degree of jaundice.

Gestational Assessment

The most widely used assessment is that described by Dubowitz and Dubowitz. Handy cards describing this assessment and the scoring system are available on application to Cow & Gate.

RESUSCITATION

Paediatric staff should be present to resuscitate babies at all deliveries involving fetal distress, where there is meconium in the liquor, malpresentation, forceps and ventouse deliveries, Caesarean section and all pre-term births.

Check Resuscitaire, paying particular attention to oxygen supply, and turn on heater.

Check other equipment:

infant laryngoscopes (have a spare);

mucus extractor;

endotracheal tubes for infants:

2·5 mm ET tubes for infants < 1·75 kg

3·0 mm ET tubes for infants 1·75–3·5 kg

3·5 mm ET tubes for infants > 3·5 kg

(occasionally 2 mm ET tubes for infants < 750 g may be required);

connections to fit ET tubes to oxygen supply (which should have a blow-off valve set at 30 cm H_2O);

suction catheters 6FG and 8FG;

syringes;

Ampoules of 8·4% $NaHCO_3$, naloxone*, adrenaline 1:1,000.

Method

Dry infant, wrap in warm dry towel/blanket, suck out

---

* Standard ampoules containing 0·4 mg/ml are recommended. Narcan Neonatal only contains 0·02 mg/ml. Only stock one or other on Resuscitaire to avoid confusion.

mouth and nose with mucus extractor, stimulate to breathe, pinching knee.

Intubation and IPPV

Intubate immediately if infant heart rate is less than 80/min and not gasping or if heart rate is around 80/min and infant is intermittently gasping. Give two static inflations lasting 2–3 seconds at peak airway pressure (PAP) 30 cm H_2O then continue IPPV at rate 30–40/min PAP 20–25 cm H_2O. Remember that infants who have been sectioned for fetal distress need intubating sooner than infants delivered by elective lower segment Caesarean section (LSCS) and so do prematurely born infants who withstand hypoxia and adapt less well to extra-uterine life than those born at term.

Problems

(i) *Intubated infant pink but won't breathe:* consider (*a*) respiratory depression, e.g. pethidine and general anaesthetic, (*b*) low arterial CO_2 resulting from over-ventilation, (*c*) possible hypoxic brain damage, (*d*) possible severe acidosis.

(ii) *Correctly intubated infant won't turn pink:* consider if there could be: (*a*) metabolic acidosis, (*b*) pneumothorax, (*c*) diaphragmatic hernia, (*d*) hypoplastic lungs, (*e*) severe hyaline membrane disease (very immature infants), (*f*) congenital heart disease (cyanotic congenital heart disease rarely presents as failure to turn pink).

(iii) *Heart rate remains below 40 per minute:* compress midsternum against vertebral column approximately 120–140 times per minute while maintaining IPPV. The use of adrenaline 1 ml of 1:10,000 (dilute 1:1,000 with normal saline) has been advocated if no heart rate is heard after several lung inflations, but the brain may have already suffered irreparable damage. If the infant is not depressed by drugs or acidosis, has no congenital abnormality and is not breathing by himself by 30–45 minutes of age, cease resuscitative measures.

(iv) *Meconium aspiration syndrome.*—In the presence of meconium-stained liquor a paediatrician should be present at delivery to:

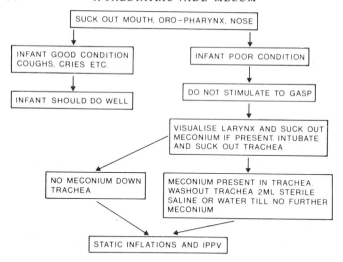

Drugs used in Resuscitation

(*a*) *Naloxone* (morphine/pethidine antagonist). Give naloxone 0·2 mg intramuscularly if estimated birth weight is more than 2 kg or 0·1 mg if below 2 kg. Intramuscularly it takes 3–4 minutes to act and the effect persists for 18 hours. Naloxone I.V. (dose 0·04 mg) acts more quickly but, as the effect wears off after 3–4 hours, give an additional dose intramuscularly at the same time.

(*b*) *Sodium bicarbonate* for correction of metabolic acidosis. Correct presumed metabolic acidosis only after taking blood for Astrup and when infant is having IPPV or is breathing adequately. Give 5–15 ml (depending on size of baby) of 8·4 per cent sodium bicarbonate slowly and with great care over a period of 10–15 minutes through a catheter or No. 1 needle into the umbilical vein.

(*c*) *Adrenaline:* 1 ml of 1:10,000 (dilute 1:1,000 with normal saline) give intracardiac if heart beat not heard (see above).

FEEDING AND FLUIDS

Well, full-term babies should be put to the breast as soon after delivery as is practicable, ideally in the delivery room.

Feeding should be not delayed in those whose weight falls below the tenth centile for gestation, the pre-term who are otherwise well and term babies who need special care. Babies should have gentle stomach washout with sterile water at body temperature using 5 ml aliquots until the fluid aspirated is clear. Following the washout give first feed as 5 per cent dextrose (5 ml under 2·0 kg, 10 ml more than 2·0 kg) and continue with milk feeds as follows:

	Well, term infants appropriate for gestation	Well, pre-term <37 weeks and small-for-dates	"Ill" pre-term and small-for-dates
Day 1	60 ml/kg/24 hours	60 ml/kg/24 hours	60 ml/kg/24 hours
Day 2	90 ml/kg/24 hours	90 ml/kg/24 hours	60 ml/kg/24 hours
Day 3	120 ml/kg/24 hours	120 ml/kg/24 hours	90 ml/kg/24 hours
Day 4	150 ml/kg/24 hours	150 ml/kg/24 hours	90 ml/kg/24 hours
Day 5	150 ml/kg/24 hours	180 ml/kg/24 hours	120 ml/kg/24 hours
Day 6	150 ml/kg/24 hours	200 ml/kg/24 hours	120 ml/kg/24 hours
Day 7	150 ml/kg/24 hours	200 ml/kg/24 hours	150 ml/kg/24 hours
Day 8	150 ml/kg/24 hours	200 ml/kg/24 hours	150 ml/kg/24 hours
			Further increase to 180 and 200 ml depends on recovery from illness.

Fluids.—Infants having I.V. fluids should have incremental increases up to a total volume intake of 150 ml/kg/24 hours as 4 per cent dextrose and 0·18 per cent saline. For details see Table X, page 61.

Add calcium and potassium supplements to the infusion after 24 hours on I.V. fluids, as calcium gluconate 1 mmol/kg/day (=4·4 ml 10 per cent calcium gluconate/kg/day) and potassium 2·5 mmol/kg/day (=1·25 ml of Strong potassium chloride solution B.P./kg/day) if blood biochemistry indicates the need.

Babies naked under phototherapy lights or radiant heaters require extra water—30 ml/kg/24 hours added to the feed to offset that lost by evaporation.

Vitamin and iron supplements.—Add vitamin and iron

supplements to babies whose birth weight < 2·5 kg from day 14 as follows:

> Abidec 1 ml daily
> Ferrous sulphate 30 mg daily
> Folic acid 1 mg daily

Add supplements to feeds after autoclaving.

Remember that very small babies can develop vitamin D deficient rickets. Check alkaline phosphatase weekly from three weeks of age in infants with a birth weight of less than 1·5 kg and, if high, increase total vitamin D intake to 1,200 units per day using calciferol.

SPECIFIC NEONATAL PROBLEMS

TEMPERATURE

After drying and wrapping in warm blankets, full-term normal infants may be handled by their parents. Delivery room and nurseries should have an ambient temperature of at least 25°C. Room temperatures for infants who are ill or small should range between 26–28°C. Ill or small babies need to be nursed in ambient temperatures corresponding to their neutral thermal range. On day 1 the appropriate temperatures for naked and fully-clothed babies are:

	1 kg	2 kg	3 kg
Unclothed (in incubators with a Perspex heat shield)	34·5–35·5	33·0–34·5	32·0–34·0°C
Clothed (in a cot with light blankets)	28·5–31·0	25·0–29·5	23·0–29·0°C

Simply putting on a bonnet and a few clothes cuts down heat loss by radiation, evaporation, convection and conduction. Ask the question "Does this infant need to be naked?" Small but relatively well babies in incubators should be clothed.

Cold infants ($<35°C$) have to be placed in ambient temperatures higher than their neutral thermal range, using overhead heater and incubator, and in larger babies a protected heating pad.

HYPOGLYCAEMIA

There may be signs such as irritability, tremulousness, twitching, convulsions, cyanotic or apnoeic attacks: hypoglycaemia may, however, be entirely asymptomatic especially in babies "at risk" or "ill".

"*At risk*" babies include the low-birth-weight, the light-for-dates, the post-mature, infants of diabetic mothers and those with temperatures of 35° or less. Starvation, e.g. surgical problems, rhesus disease, maternal tolbutamide and the Beckwith syndrome also predispose.

"*Ill babies*" would include those with perinatal hypoxia, infection or respiratory distress.

Both these groups need to be screened by using Dextrostix at birth and three-hourly for 36 hours, as well as early prophylactic feeding. If at any time values for Dextrostix fall below 1·5 mmol/l (25 mg/dl) blood glucose should be estimated and treatment started as indicated below. Blood estimations are then continued hourly until the tests show levels of 2·0 mmol/l or more.

Prevention

Infants who are designated "**at risk**" but are clinically well should have their stomachs washed out soon after birth and 5–10 ml of 5 per cent dextrose left in the stomach at the end of the procedure. This is followed by a milk feed within two hours of birth, repeated every 1–2 hours if below 2 kg or 2–3 hourly if above 2 kg according to the following schedule: 60 ml/kg 1st 24 h, then 90, 120, 150, 180 and 200 ml/kg on succeeding 24 h periods.

"**Ill**" babies need careful assessment before commencing milk feeds. Nasogastric feeding should only be attempted if the infant is well enough, otherwise peripheral I.V. infusion with 4·3 per cent dextrose in 0·18 per cent saline should be given.

Use of umbilical vein in these circumstances is hazardous.

TREATMENT OF HYPOGLYCAEMIA

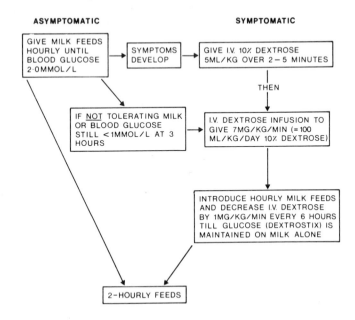

If 7 mg/kg/min dextrose (4 ml/kg/hr 10 per cent dextrose) fails to restore glucose homeostasis, increase progressively to 12 mg/kg/min and, if that fails, consider use of I.V. or I.M. hydrocortisone 5 mg/kg stat and then 1 mg/kg six-hourly. Glucagon 20 micrograms/kg can be tried even in small-for-dates (SFD) babies when there is a sudden severe fall of blood glucose that cannot be raised with I.V. dextrose. Resistant hypoglycaemia may also be the presenting sign of rare conditions as described on page 197.

OXYGEN THERAPY

Oxygen administered for any length of time should be warmed and humidified, administered via headbox and the inspired concentration measured and recorded every 30–60 minutes. PaO_2 should be maintained between 8–10 kPa which is particularly important for babies less than 36 weeks gestation. Transcutaneous measurements are not always reliable and need confirmation by arterial sampling.

RESPIRATORY DISTRESS SYNDROME

This is characterised by the onset shortly after birth of some or all of the following: tachypnoea, tachycardia, intercostal recession, sternal depression, expiratory grunt, cyanosis in air.

Causes include persistent lung fluid or minor aspiration producing transitory tachypnoea of the newborn, idiopathic respiratory distress syndrome (IRDS) due to relative pulmonary surfactant deficiency (synonymous with hyaline membrane disease), pneumothorax, pneumonia (particularly group B strep.), meconium aspiration, diaphragmatic hernia and aspiration of milk. **Remember that cold babies grunt.** Less common causes include hypoplastic lungs (Potter's syndrome), thoracic dystrophy, tracheo-oesophageal fistula, laryngeal clefts, choanal atresia, compression of trachea. Other possible causes of persistent breathlessness are heart failure and metabolic acidosis.

Management

1. Keep nasopharynx clear of mucus and milk: if aspiration suspected suck out mouth and nasopharynx.
2. Give oxygen for central cyanosis and maintain PaO_2 8–10 kPa.
3. Exclude heart failure and congenital anomaly.
4. Perform arterial Astrup to assess oxygenation and to exclude severe metabolic acidosis (capillary Astrup is adequate for pH, base excess and Pco_2 but is useless for assessing arterial oxygenation).
5. X-ray chest. Good quality films are the only means of establishing which lung pathology is causing the RDS, but handling must be minimal and the infant kept warm (transillumination may become the quickest and safest way of diagnosing a pneumothorax).
6. Pass nasogastric tube and aspirate. Set up I.V. drip with 4·3 per cent dextrose 0·18 per cent saline.
7. Correct metabolic acidosis. If base excess worse than −12 mmol/l correct base deficit slowly over 6–8 hours

(B.Wt. (kg)×0·3×base deficit = number of mmol NaHCO$_3$ to correct fully).

8. Antibiotics may have a place and if in doubt *remember that unexpected RDS babies above 36 weeks' gestation should be treated with great urgency, as group B streptococcal pneumonia can mimic IRDS perfectly.* Give benzyl penicillin I.V. or I.M. with or without gentamicin (see dose, page 94). Also remember that maternal streptococcal infection can be responsible for premature labour.

APNOEIC ATTACKS

Once breathing has been re-established, examine the baby to exclude respiratory problems (especially those following the aspiration of milk) and heart failure. Other causes include infection, hypoxia and maternal drugs. Hypoglycaemia, metabolic acidosis, hypocalcaemia and hypomagnasaemia should also be looked for. Treat recognisable disease right away and do not delay the prescription of antibiotics if infection is suspected.

Babies with apnoeic attacks, even if they are short-lived, need to be carefully supervised and monitored. Babies below 2·0 kg may need to be fed every 1–2 hours to reduce the risk of further attacks and aspiration. Repeated attacks may cease with extra oxygen but PaO$_2$ must be monitored. They may also be prevented by oral theophylline, 3 mg/kg/8-hourly. Check levels 36–48 hours after starting treatment, two hours after an oral dose, thereafter every 2–3 days depending on levels (safe level 7–15 mg/l). Alternatively give I.V. aminophylline 0·8–1·0 mg/kg/hour to maintain similar blood levels. CAUTION, if tachycardia persistently above 165/min consider reducing dose slowly. If theophylline or aminophylline are stopped suddenly, further apnoeic spells may be precipitated. Repeated attacks which fail to respond to the above measures may need CPAP or IPPV. If attacks are severe, intubation and IPPV should not be delayed.

Assisted Respiration and Transfer for Intensive Care

It is impossible to define the right time to institute CPAP or IPPV or to transfer to a newborn intensive care unit. Much depends on the size and gestation of the baby, the speed at which the disease progresses and the facilities and expertise available on site. Broadly speaking, the following rules apply:

1. CPAP may be used if baby is breathing well when arterial oxygen (PaO_2) falls below 8 kPa in 60 per cent inspired oxygen. But units that treat babies with CPAP should also have facilities for IPPV and direct measurement of arterial oxygen.

2. Babies below 2 kg which require CPAP before 24 hours are also likely to need IPPV. Transfer when inspired oxygen concentration needed to maintain colour exceeds 40 per cent if the unit does not have the experience and facilities for IPPV. Try to make such decisions early in the day.

JAUNDICE

Early Jaundice

Jaundice appearing in the first 24 hours is abnormal and haemolysis or infection must be excluded.

ABO incompatibility:
  Mother O, Baby A or B. Coombs may be slightly +ve or −ve. Send maternal blood for haemolysins.

Rhesus and other incompatibilities:
  Anti-D iso-immunoglobulin should have been detected antenatally, but anti-C, E, c, e, may not. All rhesus affected infants together with anti-Kell, anti-Duffy and other rare blood group incompatibilities will be detected by a +ve Coombs test.

Red cell abnormalities:
  Congenital spherocytosis (examine blood films and if suggestive check in parents).
  G-6-PD deficiency especially if Mediterranean, African or Asian.

Infection:
  Carry out infection screen, see page 93. In rubella, CMV or toxoplasmosis baby is often ill with enlarged liver and spleen. Total and specific IgM on infant may be helpful.

Unexplained or "Physiological" Jaundice

Appears after 48 hours and characteristically does not rise above 200 μmol/l. It may be accentuated by bruising, breast feeding and infection and usually disappears by 7–10th day of life.

Management of Hyperbilirubinaemia

Treat unconjugated non-haemolytic hyperbilirubinaemia by phototherapy or exchange transfusion according to the action lines in Fig. 2.

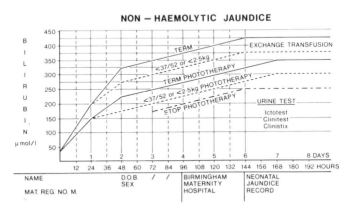

Fig. 2

Phototherapy

Keep infant warm and offset increased fluid loss from evaporation by adding 30 ml/kg per day of extra water to daily fluid intake. Protect the eyes from bright light and explain possible side-effects, i.e. skin rash and change in nature of stools to parents.

Exchange Transfusion

(a) Cross-match against infant and maternal serum (compatible rhesus negative blood should always be used in rhesus disease). Whole citrate phosphate dextrose (CPD) blood not more than five days old should be used unless infant is anaemic, when packed cells should be used for the first 80 ml/kg exchanged.

(b) Warm blood to 37°C. Overheating will cause haemolysis.

(c) Catheterise umbilical vein or artery.

(d) Keep infant warm and monitor heart by continuous ECG.

(e) Start with an "out" (5 ml from infants < 1 kg, 10 ml from larger infants). Aim to exchange twice blood volume (i.e. total 160 ml/kg) in about two hours.

(*f*) Heart rate fluctuations of more than 20 beats/min from resting value indicate the infant needs a rest. Stop the exchange until heart rate has settled.

(*g*) I.V. calcium during exchange is not necessary with CPD blood.

(*h*) Make sure you end up putting IN as much as you take OUT. **Scrupulous records are essential.**

Haemolytic Disease of the Newborn

It may present with life-threatening anaemia at birth, kernicterus hours or days later and 'late' anaemia in succeeding weeks.

At birth check cord blood for ABO and rhesus grouping, Coombs, haemoglobin, total bilirubin, and examine infant for anaemia, jaundice, oedema, liver, spleen, ascites and pleural fluid. (Note: haemoglobin level from heel prick or venous sample taken after birth may be 3–4 g/dl higher than cord samples because of fluid shift).

1. Infants who are clearly very anaemic and ill (Hb less than 7 g/dl) need urgent small exchange transfusion of not more than one volume (80 ml/kg) with 'O' Rh −ve packed cells. The second volume of the exchange should be with whole blood and may be delayed by 1–3 hours if the child did not tolerate the first volume well.

2. If haemoglobin is < 12 g/dl but infant is not seriously ill, exchange as soon as blood is cross-matched and packed. Give 1 volume packed cells followed by 1 volume whole blood: phototherapy is of secondary importance: monitor initially with 3-hourly bilirubin and 1-hourly Dextrostix.

3. If haemoglobin is greater than 12 g/dl and cord bilirubin > 85 μmol/1, check bilirubin three-hourly and give phototherapy, but may need early exchange. If cord bilirubin < 85 μmol/1 check bilirubin 4-hourly and may need phototherapy.

A bilirubin level which rises faster than 8·5 μmol/1 (0·5 mg/100 ml) per hour will usually need exchange transfusion to control it (Consult).

4. "Late Anaemia." All Coombs-positive infants should have haemoglobin prior to discharge and regularly thereafter for eight weeks. Top-up transfusion with rhesus-negative

blood (packed cells) is indicated when Hb less than 7·5 g/dl in otherwise asymptomatic infants.

Prolonged Jaundice

Jaundice persisting or presenting after 10 days of age (14 in immature baby) is abnormal. Infection, hypothyroidism, metabolic disease, alpha₁ antitrypsin deficiency, tyrosinaemia, galactosaemia and cystic fibrosis have to be excluded before the difficult differentiation between neonatal hepatitis and biliary duct atresia can be tackled. If infant is breast feeding and thriving and liver enzymes are normal, it is probably safe to assume that prolonged jaundice is associated with breast feeding and this should fade by six weeks of age. The differential diagnosis between neonatal hepatitis and biliary atresia cannot be made by biochemical tests alone. If a specific cause of hepatocellular damage cannot be identified, then in expert hands a needle biopsy of the liver will in 90 per cent of cases distinguish biliary atresia from neonatal hepatitis. Babies with biliary atresia should be operated upon by eight weeks of age.

HYPOCALCAEMIA

A low serum calcium ($< 1·7$ mmol/l) is commonly discovered in the first few days of life in the small preterm, the ill and infants of diabetic mothers, especially if they are on I.V. drips. Symptoms are uncommon. It can also follow exchange transfusion with acid citrate dextrose blood. Later in the first week symptomatic hypocalcaemia may still occasionally follow modified formula feeding. Hypocalcaemia in Asian babies may be associated with neonatal rickets. Primary hypoparathyroidism and maternal hyperparathyroidism are very rare causes.

Common symptoms are jitteriness and fits. Tetany, heart failure, generalised oedema, bradycardia and heart block are rare.

Investigations include serum calcium, phosphorus, alkaline phosphatase and magnesium. ECG if cardiac signs present. X-ray if rickets suspected. Check maternal calcium, phosphorus and alkaline phosphatase.

Treatment

(*a*) *Asymptomatic biochemical hypocalcaemia* in babies on I.V. infusions: (calcium < 1·7 mmol/1). Add calcium 1 mmol/kg/day to infusion as 10 per cent calcium gluconate (4·4 ml/kg/day). Monitor serum calcium daily. Avoid forehead veins as "tissuing" leads to pitting and scarring. Do not mix with sodium bicarbonate.

(*b*) *Symptomatic hypocalcaemia:* (calcium always < 1·5 mmol/1). Oral treatment preferable.

1. Feed on low phosphate formula or human milk;

2. Give oral calcium supplements 1 mmol/kg per 24 hours as 10 per cent calcium gluconate (4·4 ml/kg per 24 hours) or 10 per cent calcium lactate (3·1 ml/kg per 24 hours) in 4–6 divided doses;

3. Calciferol 1200 units per day orally for rickets and in resistant cases where magnesium level is normal.

Intravenous.—In severe convulsions, heart block or failure, give 0·2 ml/kg of 10 per cent calcium gluconate diluted in 4·8 ml/kg of 0·9 per cent saline slowly over 5–10 minutes I.V. Continuous ECG monitoring is necessary as heart can arrest in systole. To maintain serum calcium level continue as for "asymptomatic hypocalcaemia".

HYPOMAGNESAEMIA

This is less common than hypocalcaemia but consider it in differential diagnosis of convulsions, especially if calcium and other investigations are normal or if hypocalcaemia persists despite conventional treatment.

Treatment

If serum magnesium is below 0·4 mmol/l give oral magnesium 0·6 mmol/kg per 24 hours as 10 per cent magnesium chloride (1·2 ml/kg per 24 hours) or 10 per cent magnesium sulphate (1·5 ml/kg per 24 hours) in four divided doses for 24 hours. If parenteral route is indicated give 0·075 ml/kg of magnesium sulphate 50 per cent injection (Mg^{++} 0·15 mmol/kg) diluted in 0·3 ml/kg of water I.M. or slowly I.V. while monitoring with ECG.

CONVULSIONS

Fits may masquerade as apnoeic or cyanotic attacks, cycling movements of the limbs or abnormal mouthing. In first 48 hours perinatal hypoxia, intracranial trauma, intracranial haemorrhage and hypoglycaemia are the most likely causes. Infection, especially meningitis, must be considered at all times. Fits associated with low calcium, magnesium or sodium tend to appear later. Cortical vein thrombosis resulting from polycythaemia or dehydration should be considered.

Management

Control immediate convulsion(s) and carry out infection and metabolic screen.

Treatment

(1) Control fit with diazepam I.V. 0·3 mg/kg (be ready to intubate if apnoea results) or if vein is not immediately accessible give 1 ml of paraldehyde I.M. if over 2·5 kg or 0·3 ml/kg if under 2·5 kg.

(2) Prevent further attacks with phenobarbitone 10 mg/kg I.M. 12-hourly to *total* dose of 60–90 mg/kg. Then stop or maintain 2·5–5·0 mg/kg 12-hourly. If fits continue in spite of adequate treatment and normal investigations, give 25 mg pyridoxine I.V. as a therapeutic trial.

THE ILL BABY

The newborn, especially if preterm, may rapidly deteriorate and just "look ill" when suffering from a variety of disturbances, be they infection (bacterial or viral), cerebral injury or haemorrhage, other blood loss, cardiac or renal failure, or metabolic disease. The symptoms are protean and range from a slight change in behaviour or feeding pattern, instability of temperature and vomiting to sudden collapse.

Most, if not all, of the problems described below come within the differential diagnosis and it is frequently necessary to carry out an infection and metabolic screen in these circumstances. The investigations listed below are usually indicated, modified in the light of common sense.

Infection Screen

Ear, umbilical, nose and throat swabs, WBC and differential, PCV, blood culture. Suprapubic bladder aspiration. Lumbar puncture. Chest (and sometimes abdominal) X-rays. Viral studies. IgM.

Metabolic Screen

Astrup. Electrolytes and urea. Blood glucose, calcium and magnesium. Amino acids in blood and urine in selected cases.

INFECTIONS

(*a*) **Antepartum and Intrapartum: Premature rupture of membranes.**—If the membranes have been ruptured for more than 18 hours, infection should be suspected. The primary site is in the lung proceeding often to meningitis. Carry out an infection screen and Astrup and note that a neutrophil count below $2 \cdot 0 \times 10^9$/l or an increasing metabolic acidosis point to infection.

Treat all ill and breathless babies with antibiotics (see Table XV) and consider treatment in the immature and those who have had instrumental, difficult or hypoxic deliveries. Watch carefully.

(*b*) **The ill probably infected baby.**—Carry out infection and metabolic screen and note that after the third day of life an absolute neutrophil count greater than $7 \cdot 0 \times 10^9$/l suggests bacterial infection. If an alternative diagnosis does not emerge immediately start treatment with systemic antibiotics I.M. or I.V. Start with either penicillin and gentamicin or cefuroxime, although the latter is ineffective against *Pseudomonas aeruginosa* and *Listeria monocytogenes*. Add metronidazole (protect from light) if anaerobic infection is suspected. If CSF contains more than 20 WBC/cu mm (20×10^6/l), meningitis is likely and chloramphenicol should be given I.V. until the culture has been reported. Gentamicin does not pass the blood brain barrier.

(*c*) **Superficial infection:**

> *Skin, nares, umbilicus and nail folds* are primary sites of Staphylococcal infection. Swab, isolate and barrier nurse with mother. Cross-infection is best confirmed by bacteriophage typing and prevented by careful hand washing

TABLE XV

ANTIBIOTICS—DOSES, ROUTES AND FREQUENCY OF ADMINISTRATION ACCORDING TO GESTATION AND POSTNATAL AGE

Antibiotic	Individual Dose	Gestation					
		Less than 37 weeks			More than 37 weeks		
		Postnatal age	Timing	Route	Postnatal age	Timing	Route
Ampicillin Benzylpenicillin Flucloxacillin	30 mg/kg 50 mg/kg 30 mg/kg	<7 days 7–14 days 14 days+	12-hourly 8-hourly 6-hourly	I.M./I.V. I.M./I.V. I.M./I.V.	as before		
Carbenicillin	100 mg/kg	<7 days 7 days+	12-hourly 8-hourly	I.V. I.V.	<7 days 7 days+	8-hourly 6-hourly	I.V. I.V.
Cefuroxime	30 mg/kg	<7 days 7 days+	12-hourly 8-hourly	I.M./I.V. I.M./I.V.	<4 days 4 days+	12-hourly 8-hourly	I.M./I.V. I.M./I.V.
Chloramphenicol	12·5 mg/kg	0–4 weeks 4 weeks+	12-hourly 8-hourly	I.V. I.V.	0–14 days 14 days+	12-hourly 8-hourly	I.V. I.V.
Gentamicin	2·5 mg/kg	<7 days 7 days+	12-hourly 8-hourly	I.M./I.V. I.M./I.V.	as before		
		Babies < 1000 g <14 days 14 days+	18-hourly 12-hourly	I.M./I.V. I.M./I.V.			
Metronidazole	7·5 mg/kg	8-hourly I.V. probably for all gestations.					

and the routine use of hexachlorophene powder, especially in the axillae and groins, as well as a strict routine for the care of the cord. Single skin lesions may be dried with chlorhexidine in alcohol but, if spreading or infection present in other sites, treat with flucloxacillin I.M. then orally after swab has been taken. Staphylococci are often isolated from the nose of babies with snuffles. Treat symptoms with 0·5 per cent ephedrine in saline nose drops but if blockage or discharge persist use flucloxacillin I.M. then orally.

Eyes. Send swabs from all discharging eyes directly and immediately to the laboratory in transport medium. If profuse, make smear at cot side as well. Discharge can often be cleared with regular 2-hourly irrigations of tepid sterile water. Treat persistent discharge with chloramphenicol 0·5 per cent eye drops every 1–2 hours and, if this fails, consider chlamydia or gonococcal infections. (Gonococcal ophthalmia may be misdiagnosed if a smear is not taken to demonstrate intracellular diplococci. The gonococcus is notoriously difficult to culture—hence transport medium.) Treat chlamydial infections with tetracycline eye ointment and two weeks' oral erythromycin.

Mouth and groins. Oral thrush may be treated with oral nystatin 100,000 units before feeds. It also often infects the groins of small babies, being recognised by site and the presence of satellite lesions. Expose to keep the area dry and apply nystatin or miconazole cream: if persistent, give treatment by mouth as well.

Anaemia, Shock, Haemorrhage

Anaemia and haemorrhagic shock at or shortly after birth may result from blood loss into the maternal circulation (fetomaternal bleed), damage to the placenta or cord, haemorrhage into the muscles in breech delivery and into other tissues in difficult instrumental deliveries. Identical twins are at particular risk of bleeding one into the other and in such cases the anaemia may be acute or chronic. Haemorrhagic shock a few days after birth following a rupture of an abdominal viscus may be associated with organ enlargement and bluish staining around the umbilicus or groin, but such signs are inconstant. Ultrasound may help in the detection of collections of blood. Investigations include Hb, blood grouping, Coombs, coagulation status. Take blood from mother for Kleihauer and blood grouping.

Management.—If baby is anaemic and shocked, treat with an immediate transfusion of O Rh −ve blood or, if not available, restore circulation with plasma. Give vitamin K_1 1 mg I.M. to prevent hypoprothrombinaemia. Use fresh frozen plasma 10 ml/kg if bleeding persists. Purpura and bleeding from disseminated intravascular coagulation may occur in any ill baby. Effective correction of the primary condition is the most useful treatment but an exchange transfusion with fresh whole blood may be helpful in the interim.

PLETHORA AND POLYCYTHAEMIA

This occurs in infants who have been malnourished or chronically hypoxic *in utero*, in an identical twin and in the baby of the diabetic mother. The viscosity of blood rises rapidly when venous PCV $>$ 70 per cent. Management depends on platelet and coagulation status and should anticipate development of neurological and respiratory symptoms. Unfortunately, the interpretation of results and the management is complex and at present beyond the scope of this section. Nevertheless, if dilution exchange is to be carried out use fresh frozen plasma or plasma to lower PCV to 60 per cent (volume to be exchanged in ml) =

$$\frac{\text{PCV measured} - \text{PCV desired} \times 80 \times \text{B.Wt in kg}}{\text{PCV measured}}$$

GASTRO-INTESTINAL SYMPTOMS

Hydramnios.—Exclude oesophageal and duodenal atresia. Pass wide-bore catheter through the mouth into the oesophagus; a mucus extractor is ideal. If the catheter's progress is arrested or loops back, atresia is likely. An X-ray may show the radio-opaque catheter coiled in the upper pouch. In suspected cases nothing should be given by mouth until the condition has been excluded. Duodenal atresia is a less common cause of hydramnios.

Vomiting.—This is common in the first 24 hours when vomit usually contains swallowed blood, mucus or meconium. One or two stomach washouts may be needed before vomiting ceases. If it persists, is bile-stained or associated with abdominal distension and delay in passage of meconium, exclude intestinal obstruction with supine and erect X-rays of abdomen. In babies with a low obstruction and well enough to stand the procedure, a lateral film taken after the baby has been held head down for 5–10 minutes will show whether air has entered the colon and rectum. Once intestinal obstruction has been confirmed make sure that vitamin K has been given and maternal blood (needed for cross-matching) is transferred with the baby and the consent form to the surgical unit. Vomiting may also occur with cerebral irritation, hiatus hernia, rectal mucus plug (meconium plug syndrome) or ganglion-blocking drugs given to the mother. It may also be a symptom of infection and congenital adrenal hyperplasia, while in the second week pyloric stenosis has to be considered.

Delay in the Passage of Meconium beyond 24 Hours

Hirschsprung's disease and cystic fibrosis may need to be excluded in a healthy term baby, but the symptom is common in ill and/or immature babies. Some newborn babies who become distended and show other signs of intestinal obstruction eventually pass a "mucus plug"—which appears to be a cast of an undistended colon. Once passed, normal bowel function is then established. This condition, otherwise known as the meconium plug syndrome, may initially resemble Hirschsprung's disease and, in some cases, may be the first sign of the condition. It may need to be formally excluded by rectal biopsy if subsequent bowel function is suspect. Cystic fibrosis must be ruled out by sweat test at six weeks of age.

Necrotising Enterocolitis (NEC)

It most often develops in immature babies towards the end of, or after, the first week of life and may be sporadic or epidemic in occurrence. In the mildest form there is a little blood and mucus with loose stools and little or no systemic disturbance. At the other end of the spectrum sudden abdominal distension and tenderness and the passage of blood, mucus and intestinal mucosa herald a fulminating illness.

Management by Degree of Severity of Illness

(1) *Mild:* Blood and mucus passed P.R. but baby relatively well and there is no abdominal distension or tenderness. Isolate baby and barrier nurse. Stop further admissions or transfers out of "infected cubicle" from which it came. Culture faeces: check haemoglobin, WBC and differential and platelets, supine and erect X-ray of abdomen. Stop all feeds and start I.V. Watch carefully and review frequently with view to early antibiotic treatment.

(2) *Moderate:* Baby is unwell and in addition there is abdominal distension. Group and cross-match baby. Stop all feeds and maintain hydration with I.V. fluids. Treat with benzyl penicillin, gentamicin and metronidazole. Inform surgeons. Watch and review frequently. Re-introduce graded feeds with care once all signs have abated.

(3) *Severe:* Baby is seriously ill. X-ray: look particularly for signs of gas under the diaphragm and/or in the branches of the portal vein and INVOLVE SURGEONS, irrespective of results. Repeated X-rays at 6-hourly intervals may be needed to determine progression and appropriate time for surgery if necessary. Look for disseminated intravascular coagulation (DIC). Medical management as in (2), including vigorous management of "shock" with plasma expanders. Indications for laparotomy:
   (*a*) progressive deterioration despite resuscitation,
   (*b*) perforation,
   (*c*) progressive distension and/or extension of pneumatoses.

Outbreaks of NEC may occur in an intensive care unit and can only be stopped by partial or complete closure of the unit.

VIRAL INFECTIONS IN LATE PREGNANCY AND THE NEONATE

Cytomegalovirus.—Cervical infection rises to around 10 per cent (USA) in late pregnancy; transplacental infection is uncommon. Risk of infecting the baby or of cross-infection is small. If baby becomes infected there is negligible risk of cross-infection. Nevertheless, if in intensive care nursery, isolate.

Herpes simplex virus (HSV).—Cervical or vaginal herpes infection is three times more common in pregnancy, but intra-uterine infections remain very rare. Risk of neonatal infection is 10 per cent if mother has cytological, serological or clinical evidence of genital infection (primary or recurrent) at 32 weeks, but this rises to 40 per cent if infection is present at delivery unless the infant is delivered by Caesarean section within four hours from rupture of membranes. Immunoglobulin after birth is of doubtful benefit. Idoxuridine may be useful treatment. Isolate. Facial herpes in attendants has very low risk to mother or to baby. Treat early lesions with idoxuridine.

Measles.—Only 10 per cent parturient women are susceptible. If measles infects the mother late in pregnancy or after birth give "normal" immunoglobulin to baby. Maternal antibody passes placenta.

Mumps.—No passive protection. If maternal infection takes place around birth protect baby with "normal" immunoglobulin.

Rubella.—If suspected in newborn, isolate. Confirm diagnosis by checking maternal immune status at booking and test for specific IgM in baby and maternal/infant antibody titres. Ensure that attendants are immune. Baby remains infectious for at least six months. Non-immune mothers should be offered immunisation in puerperium as a routine.

Varicella.—Maternal varicella within the four days before delivery or after, presents a serious danger to baby. Separate mother and baby and isolate both. Give Zoster immunoglobulin (ZIG) 0·1 ml/kg at birth. If unobtainable use "normal" immunoglobulin 1 ml/kg but it may only modify disease. Ensure baby is nursed by immune staff. If maternal varicella appears earlier than five days before birth, the baby is usually infected but, due to passage of maternal antibodies, is safe. No specific action is needed: keep mother and baby together.

Herpes zoster in the mother is unlikely to give rise to fetal or neonatal infection. Isolate mother with baby and nurse with immune staff. Varicella zoster antibody crosses placenta to give protection.

Hepatitis A or B presenting with jaundice in late pregnancy or labour.—Management at birth: Isolate mother and baby separately until results reported upon.

Results	Action
Mother hepatitis B +ve Core antibody +ve Surface antigen +ve or −ve Baby hepatitis B −ve	Give baby hepatitis B immunoglobulin and reunite with mother on isolation ward. Blood and urine samples from mother remain a biohazard
Mother hepatitis B +ve Baby hepatitis B +ve	Reunite on isolation ward. Urine and blood specimens remain a biohazard
Mother hepatitis A +ve Baby hepatitis A −ve	Give baby "normal" immunoglobulin and reunite with mother. Remain on isolation ward.
Mother hepatitis A +ve Baby hepatitis A +ve	Reunite mother and baby. Remain on isolation ward

Hepatitis B antigen +ve (HB$_s$Ag) mothers. (Usually recognised to be carriers on pregnancy screening.)

Management at birth.—Keep mother and baby together and allow breast feeding. Blood specimens are a BIO-HAZARD.

Screening of pregnant women for hepatitis B antigen (HB$_s$Ag) is routinely carried out through the Blood Transfusion Service (BTS) in some areas at the same time as blood grouping and antibodies are checked. Blood from women carriers so detected is a BIOHAZARD in pregnancy and labour, but mother and baby should, nevertheless, be kept together after birth and breast feeding allowed. Hepatitis B infection and the antigen +ve state is found in all races but is more commonly found in mothers from the developing world. The long-term risks to the baby are very small and some babies, particularly Chinese, may become antigen +ve in due course.

MATERNAL DRUGS AND BREAST FEEDING

Presumed safe	*Doubtful*	*Contra-indicated*
antihistamines	aminophylline/	anti-neoplastic agents
aspirin (low dose)	theophylline	chloramphenicol*
barbiturates (low dose)	gentamicin	co-trimoxazole**
benzodiazepines (low	aspirin (high dose)	ergot and ergotamine
dose)	barbiturates (high dose)	gold salts*
bulk laxatives	benzodiazepines (high	indomethacin
cephalosporins	dose)	iodides*
clindamycin	beta-blockers	lithium
codeine	carbamazepine	nalidixic acid
dextropropoxyphene	carbimazole*	nitrofurantoin**
digoxin	chloral	oestrogens (high dose)
erythromycin	co-trimoxazole	phenindione
flufenamic acid	corticosteroids	phenylbutazone*
folic acid	danthron (Dorbanex)	reserpine*
heparin	diuretics	sulphonamides**
ibuprofen	ethambutol	tetracyclines*
insulins	hypoglycaemics	
iron	isoniazid	
ketoprofen	meprobamate	
lincomycin	oestrogens (low dose)	
mefenamic acid	phenothiazines (high dose)	
methyldopa	propantheline	
metronidazole	senna	
nitrofurantoin	sodium valproate	
paracetamol	sulphonamides	
penicillins	thiouracils*	
pentazocine	thyroxine	
phenothiazines	vitamins A and D (high	
progestogens	dose)	
sodium cromoglycate	warfarin	
tricyclic antidepressants		
vitamin B group		
vitamin C		

* Theoretical risk.

**Possibility of haemolytic anaemia if baby is G-6-PD deficient.

For identification of trade-named drugs, use MIMS or Data Sheet Compendium.

From lists produced jointly by the Trent and West Midlands Drug Information Service. For further information contact Good Hope Hospital, Sutton Coldfield. Tel: (021) 378 2211.

G.M.D.
J.I.

[NOTES]

V
INFECTIONS

PYREXIA OF UNCERTAIN ORIGIN

A pyrexia of uncertain origin often has an infectious basis. Some of the conditions responsible are examined in this section but it is not intended to provide a comprehensive list or to discuss the non-infective conditions such as malignancy, inflammatory bowel disease or the collagen diseases which may present with fever.

The history must include inquiry for contact with specific infectious fevers and recent travel abroad: with children in or from tropical areas exotic disease must be seriously considered. It should also be remembered that certain diseases, such as measles, assume a more malignant and confusing picture in dark-skinned races.

In an ill child without localising signs the following tests are essential: blood, stool and urine microscopy and culture (supra-pubic aspiration in an infant), white cell count and a chest radiograph. A lumbar puncture may also be indicated subject to the proviso on page 125. In a child who has recently returned from abroad, malaria, enteric infections, T.B. and hepatitis have to be excluded even though they may present with misleading signs such as pneumonia, diarrhoea, constipation, fits, coma or anaemia. "Viral" disease is a common cause of PUO but laboratory diagnosis may be difficult or delayed. Roseola infantum falls into this group (see below).

Malaria

Malaria should be considered in any sick child who may have been exposed to infection and who presents with fever, anaemia, with or without shock, respiratory, gastro-intestinal or neurological signs or symptoms.

Convulsions or coma suggest *P. falciparum* infection causing *cerebral malaria* and immediate specific and anticonvulsant treatment is necessary. Occasional presentation in medical shock (*algid malaria*) requires urgent expansion of plasma volume as well as specific therapy. Examine thick and thin films, blood for haemoglobin and cross-matching should be taken. Treat at once with specific therapy as follows:

> chloroquine 10 mg/kg stat
> 5 mg/kg 6 hours later
> 5 mg/kg 24 hours later
> Repeat 5 mg/kg 24 hours later

and by blood transfusion if necessary. (Notifiable disease in U.K.)

Plasmodium vivax is the form of malaria most frequently acquired in India. *P. falciparum* is more common in those who come from Africa, South America and the Far East. The prophylactic administration of antimalarials does not exclude the diagnosis because (*a*) of the occurrence of drug resistant *P. falciparum*, (*b*) some patients fail to continue prophylaxis for 4–6 weeks on their arrival in the U.K., (*c*) prophylactic antimalarials do not affect the exoerythrocytic liver cycle of *P. vivax* malaria.

In Africa chloroquine resistance is rare (only reported in East Africa in 1980) but there are strains resistant to proguanil and pyrimethamine; strains of *P. falciparum* resistant to chloroquine, proguanil and pyrimethamine are widespread in S. America, Asia and the Far East (including 75 per cent of the strains in Thailand).

The treatment of choice for chloroquine-resistant *P. falciparum* is quinine followed by a combination of sulfadoxine and pyrimethamine (Fansidar). The advice of an infectious diseases expert is desirable before treating falciparum malaria acquired outside Africa.

The liver phase of *P. vivax* and *ovale* can be eliminated with primaquine but this should not be given before excluding G-6-PD deficiency.

Prophylaxis.—*P. vivax* is susceptible to all prophylactic agents. Chloroquine is suitable in areas where *P. falciparum* remains sensitive to this agent (see above). Proguanil (Paludrine) is safe for individuals with G-6-PD deficiency but will not prevent infection with resistant strains. Maloprim (pyrimethamine combined with dapsone) is suitable for short visits to regions in which chloroquine-resistant *P. falciparum* occurs. Prophylaxis should commence one week before departure and continue for 4–6 weeks after returning.

Typhoid may not show such severe constitutional symptoms as in an adult. Irregular pyrexia, cough, disturbed mental state and abdominal distension, followed by diarrhoea, splenomegaly and rose spots should lead to blood and stool culture, and serological tests. Chloramphenicol is the drug of choice in the acute stage, while ampicillin is useful in the treatment of carriers.

Tuberculosis

Infections with *Mycobacterium tuberculosis* should always be considered in the differential diagnosis. When it has already spread through the blood stream presentation may be bizarre. BEWARE Mantoux 1:1,000 which may be negative if patient is severely ill or in the early course of the disease and temporarily after measles. Examine exudates, faeces, urine or gastric washings if appropriate for *M. tuberculosis*. Biopsy or operation may occasionally be needed to confirm diagnosis.

An *opportunistic* mycobacterium, e.g. *Avium intracellulare*, may also produce lymph node enlargement and cold abscesses, especially in the cervical region; this is histologically indistinguishable from human/bovine T.B. but the Mantoux test is negative. Specific skin testing reagents to these species can be obtained in the U.K. through the Public Health Laboratory Service. T.B. is notifiable.

Hepatitis A (Infective Hepatitis)

Fever is a presenting sign and jaundice is uncommon in childhood. Its appearance heralds the disappearance of the virus from the stool so the risk of cross-infection becomes small. Serological tests now assist in the diagnosis.

Hepatitis B

Is very rare in childhood but is a problem for the neonate (see page 99).

Meningitis

Must be suspected in any acutely ill child, especially in the newborn period. The presence of an upper respiratory tract infection does not exclude its coexistence. Purpura is suggestive of meningococcaemia. Moderate pleocytosis or equivocal CSF changes may require the child to be treated especially if under a year or if previous antibiotics given. Review is then needed after culture and CSF chemistry reported upon. For causative organisms and treatment see page 254. Notifiable disease.

Roseola Infantum

Is thought to be viral in aetiology and is characterised by irritability and high fever for 3–4 days, often with no other abnormal physical signs. The fever falls by crisis, when a macular or maculo-papular rash appears on trunk and spreads, but this fades within 24 hours. The rash may be mistaken for an allergy to anti-microbial agents and must be differentiated from that of rubella and measles.

Herpes Simplex

High fever at onset of primary illness and before appearance of vesicles is usual. For keratitis give idoxuridine drops $0\cdot1$ per cent into conjunctival sac once-hourly by day and twice-hourly by night. Extensive superficial skin lesions can be treated with idoxuridine in dimethylsulphoxide. For maternal genital herpetic infection see newborn section, page 99.

CONTROL OF MEASLES IN HOSPITAL

The primary case is infectious during the prodromal phase; virus can be identified by immunofluorescence of naso-pharyngeal secretions and the immune state of contacts can be determined by fluorescent antibody techniques. If test is not available unimmunised contacts without a history of measles are "at risk", therefore discharge home within the week if possible. Isolate unimmunised contacts on the 8th day after the primary case was first thought to be infectious until the 16th day after last known contact (extend to 21 days in those given gammaglobulin).

Specific measles gammaglobulin should be given to patients within 7–10 days of exposure if there is severe congenital heart defect, T.B. or cystic fibrosis, and to those receiving cytotoxic or steroid therapy or who are otherwise immuno-compromised.

Measles vaccine should be offered to non-immune contacts who are over one year of age, provided there are no contra-indications and parents consent, as the disease may still be modified at this stage.

CONTROL OF CHICKENPOX IN HOSPITAL

Whenever a case is detected notify the Control of Infection Officer. Isolate or discharge the primary case.

All contacts, including those at the hospital school, should be identified. Assume those without a definite past history of

INCUBATION PERIOD AND DURATION OF ISOLATION OF HOSPITALISED PATIENTS

	Incubation	Isolation of the Infected Person
Chickenpox (Varicella)	10–21 days (14–15 days usually)	Until one week after the appearance of the rash or 4 days after last crop.
*Diphtheria	1–6 days	Until two consecutive negative swabs from nose and throat have been obtained.
*Enteric group	3–23 days	Until three consecutive negative stools off treatment.
*Infectious hepatitis (Hepatitis A)	15–40 days	7 days.
*Measles (Morbilli)	12–14 days (8–11 days to catarrhal stage)	7 days from the date of appearance of the rash. Patient is infective even in the prodromal phase.
Meningococcal meningitis	2 days—prolonged	For three days from commencement of antibacterial agents (see page 254).
Mumps (Epidemic Parotitis)	14–28 days (17–18 days usually)	9 days after onset of swelling.
*Poliomyelitis	5–21 days (7–14 days probably usual)	Until stool negative for polio virus.
Rubella	14–19 days (17–18 days usually)	7 days from onset of rash.
*Scarlet fever	2–5 days	For not less than 3 days following commencement of chemotherapy.
*Pertussis	7–14 days to catarrhal stage. A further 7–14 days to paroxysmal stage	For three weeks from onset of paroxysmal cough.

At risk (quarantine) time: Add 2 days to incubation period.
* Notifiable disease in U.K.

PARASITIC INFECTIONS

Parasites in the following list are either endemic in Britain (†) or are so widespread abroad that they are likely to be seen in immigrants or travellers. There are many others more localised geographically. Infestation with several worms at one time is common.

Those helminthic infestations which at some stage are particularly associated with an eosinophilia are marked with an asterisk (*).

Parasite	Diagnosis	Treatment (details see Chapter XI under individual drugs)	Special Features
(a) HELMINTHS **Nematodes** (round worms) Enterobius vermicularis† (thread worm)	Ova on perianal skin. (Sellotape slides)	Piperazine+senna (Pripsen) Mebendazole or thiabendazole	Very common. Perianal pruritus or symptomless.
Ascaris lumbricoides† (common round worm)	Ova in stools.	Piperazine (Antepar) Piperazine+senna (Pripsen) Mebendazole. Thiabendazole.	Resembles earthworm. Loeffler's syndrome.
Trichuris trichiura †* (whipworm)	Ova in stools.	Thiabendazole. Mebendazole.	May cause bloody diarrhoea or rectal prolapse.
Ankylostoma duodenale* Necator americanus (hookworm)	Ova in stools.	Bephenium (Alcopar). Mebendazole. Thiabendazole.	Common in immigrants; often causes serious blood loss (iron & protein).
Toxocara spp.†* (dog and cat round worms)	Serological tests. Histology, eye, liver and lung.	Thiabendazole.	Visceral larva migrans; history of close contact with puppies; pica.
Trichinella spiralis†*	Serological tests. Muscle biopsy (e.g. deltoid).	Thiabendazole.	History of eating raw pork sausages; fever, myalgia, orbital oedema.
Strongyloides stercoralis†*	Larvae excreted intermittently.	Thiabendazole.	Pneumonic signs; diarrhoea, abdominal pain.
Cestodes (tape worms) Taenia saginata† (beef tape worm)	Segments in stools.	Niclosamide (Yomesan).	No risk of cysticercosis.

PARASITIC INFECTIONS—*(Continued)*

Parasite	Diagnosis	Treatment	Special Features
Hymenolepis nana	Ova in stools.	Niclosamide (Yomesan).	Common in Asians. Usually symptomless.
Echinococcus granulosus (*hydatid*)	Clinical Serology. Scolices and hooklets in surgical material (hydatid "sand").	Surgical; symptomatic.	History of contact with dogs in sheep-farming areas.
(b) PROTOZOA **Entamoeba histolytica**[†]	Vegetative amoeba in dysenteric stool immediately after passing. Cysts in formed stool in carrier or case of amoebic abscess. Serology.	Metronidazole.	Most cases in patients previously resident in the tropics. Six consecutive negative stool specimens must be obtained before a patient can be considered cured.
Giardia lamblia[†]	Cysts and flagellates in fresh loose stool and duodenal specimens. Cysts in formed stool.	Metronidazole for 5-day course (dosage p. 259).	Chronic diarrhoea and malabsorption.
Toxoplasma	Positive Dye Tests and C.F.T. occur in 20–40% of "normal adults", at titres of 1/8–1/128 and in 1% at 1/256. Even a low titre signifies past infection. Fetal titre may exceed maternal in passive immunisation. IgG of maternal origin has a three-week half-life. Therefore repeat maternal and fetal titres at six weeks.	Pyrimethamine and Sulphadimidine. 12-day course (dosage see p. 263).	Neonatal hepatitis, micro- or hydrocephalus, retinitis, uveitis or microphthalmia. Ocular toxoplasmosis: usually congenital and sole lesion. Seen relatively late with visual problem when primary lesion inactive and positive dye test titres in normal range. Acquired toxoplasmosis: meningoencephalitis or pseudo-glandular fever.

chickenpox or those in whom fluorescent antibody tests show no immunity to herpes zoster to be at risk. If possible these should be discharged home forthwith. The non-immune ward staff should be identified, prevented from treating immuno-compromised patients during the "at risk" period and, if possible, transferred to an area of the hospital where all patients are immune. Each contact who cannot be discharged home must be segregated for the time it has been calculated infection could appear. In hospital, contact is usually brief, with secondary cases almost all developing vesicles between the 14th and 18th day, but they are infectious for at least four days before this. Calculate dates of exposure assuming primary case to have been infective for four days before rash and isolate from 10th day of first exposure to 21 days after last contact.

Non-immune patients readmitted during the "at risk" period should be segregated, but new patients who have not been in contact and without past history may be safely admitted to the ward.

Immunocompromised patients should be given specific herpes zoster immunoglobulin (ZIG) obtainable from the Public Health Laboratory Service. This may only modify the disease and not prevent further spread in the ward. Neonates should also receive immunoglobulin.

Staff with herpes zoster infection should not care for children.

IMMUNISATION

Timing and Contra-indications

Rubella

All teenage girls should receive rubella vaccine even though serology would show that 80 per cent are immune in the U.K. Do not give during pregnancy. Administer postnatally to mothers shown to be serologically negative.

Embryopathy risk in maternal rubella is 50 per cent in the first month falling to a low level in the fourth month. Precise history of specific contact and presence of antibody within the incubation period proves past infection. Interpretation depends on precise history and serial titres. Gammaglobulin even in high dosage offers very little protection and therefore therapeutic abortion should be considered. For fetal rubella see page 99.

For fetal rubella see page 99.

SUGGESTED IMMUNISATION SCHEDULE

(Avoid intramuscular injections in children with bleeding disorders.) See below for contra-indications to pertussis and measles vaccination.

Age	Vaccine
Newborn	BCG (Recent family history of tuberculosis or immigrant children at risk. Assess nodule at 6/52)
3 months	Diphtheria, tetanus, whooping cough, poliomyelitis: 1st dose*
5 months	Diphtheria, tetanus, whooping cough, poliomyelitis: 2nd dose
9 months	Diphtheria, tetanus, whooping cough, poliomyelitis: 3rd dose
13 months	Measles
School entry	Diphtheria, tetanus, poliomyelitis: 4th dose
10–13 years	BCG if tuberculin negative
11–14 years	Rubella (all girls)
School leaving	Tetanus, poliomyelitis: 5th dose.

* In children born prematurely commence primary immunisation at age equivalent to three months after expected birth date.

Pertussis Immunisation

Cerebral reactions are rare. Immunisation should be deferred during febrile illness and it is contra-indicated in infants with an existing CNS disorder, a history of irritability persisting over 48 hours at birth, a family history (parents and other siblings) of CNS disorder or epilepsy, a possible cerebral reaction or serious local reaction to previous dose. A family history of eczema or allergy is *not* a contra-indication.

Measles Vaccination

Contra-indicated if child has known allergy to one of the specific antibiotics used in preparing the vaccine, active T.B., steroid and cytotoxic therapy, malignancy and immune deficiencies. In children with chronic chest or heart disease, previous history of convulsions or parental history of epilepsy, delay vaccination beyond two years or give measles immunoglobulin simultaneously into the other arm. Defer during febrile illnesses and for three months after transfusion of blood products.

TETANUS PROPHYLAXIS

1. Active Immunisation

Surgical toilet of the wound is of prime importance. In addition adsorbed tetanus toxoid should be given if the child has received an incomplete course of immunisation or has not received a booster within the last five years.

Inform the patient's general practitioner, suggesting a complete course of active immunisation in those who have not previously been immunised.

2. Passive Immunisation

Category A. If the wound is clean, non-penetrating with negligible tissue damage and less than 6 hours old, antitoxin is not usually recommended.

Category B. If the wound is more serious or treatment is delayed treat initially as under Item 1. A dose of human tetanus antitoxin should be given in the opposite limb to that in which tetanus toxoid was given. A dose of tetanus antitoxin should also be given to those children whose immune status is unknown and in those who received an incomplete course or a booster over 10 years ago.

Immunisation for Travel

The legal requirements as well as the risk of contracting an infectious disease vary from one country to another. (Seek expert advice if needed.) The need for the following action should be considered. Immunisation against yellow fever, cholera and typhoid, globulin against hepatitis and prophylactic antimalarials.

In some areas of the world the risk of contracting polio, diphtheria, tetanus, measles and T.B. is significant. Immunisation is recommended.

R.H.G.

VI
PAEDIATRIC EMERGENCIES

A rapid history and examination of the seriously ill child should precede emergency treatment either in the admission room or in the ward. The parents must be asked to wait.

Once the initial treatment has been started the parents will be available to give a fuller history which may well be of the utmost importance regarding specific therapy in the early stages. Proper recording of temperature (low-reading if necessary), pulse, respiration and weight must be made. For advice on fluids and diet of ill children, see under section "Sick Children", page 25.

DEHYDRATION

Depending on the cause, symptoms may be diarrhoea, vomiting, refusal to feed or polyuria leading to apathy and coma.

Signs are loss of skin turgor, sunken fontanelle and eyeballs and circulatory failure. Factual evidence of recent loss of weight may be available from a clinic weight card.

Differential Diagnosis

1. **Gastro-enteritis of infancy.**—Fulminating cases may present before diarrhoea occurs. Rectal examination may produce the obvious evidence of a projectile watery stool and auscultation of abdomen may show either increased bowel sounds or the almost complete silence of ileus.

More commonly vomiting and diarrhoea occurs in infants with a gradual onset and less severity. Such babies if under 5 per cent dehydrated can often be treated at home with oral replacement of fluid loss with "clear" fluids.

The basic treatment of gastro-enteritis is one of fluid replacement and graded feeds (see also page 53). Cases in hospital should be isolated. Antibiotics should be reserved for the treatment of gastro-intestinal infections caused by *Salmonella typhi* and *paratyphi*, other Salmonella infections with associated septicaemia, shigellae other than *S. sonnei*, *Campylobacter jejuni* and parasitic diseases. Antibiotic treatment of bacterial gastro-enteritis in the neonate is also recommended. Antibiotics are not usually helpful or recom-

117

mended in mild gastro-intestinal infections, especially as the carriage of the causative bacterium is sometimes prolonged. Oral rehydration with "clear" fluids is the essential treatment provided the child is not in circulatory failure. The simpler the treatment the better, especially if it is to be carried out at home. Four per cent dextrose and 0·18 per cent saline from an intravenous bottle may be given orally, or commercially available glucose-electrolyte sachets prescribed (e.g. Diora-lyte) and dissolved in water, provided the mother can be upon to make it up accurately. Unless the salt can be rigorously controlled there will be an unacceptable risk of hypertonic dehydration (see p. 55).

The infant should be offered small amounts frequently (even hourly, if necessary) to provide a fluid intake of up to 180 ml per kg for the first 24 hours. If vomiting persists or the stools do not abate in frequency and dehydration increases then admission to hospital for intravenous therapy (p. 53) will be needed.

Usually after 24 hours the clinical condition improves and the child will be able to tolerate quarter-strength formula feeds which can be strengthened daily to half, three-quarters and then full strength. It is dangerous to use diphenoxylate (Lomotil) or loperamide (Imodium) for the control of acute diarrhoea in children.

2. **Other acute infections with anorexia and fever.**—E.g. bronchiolitis, otitis media, pyelonephritis or meningitis. Diar-rhoea and vomiting may also occur in association with these conditions.

3. The frequency of *other causes* varies with the age of the child. E.g. diabetes mellitus, adrenal insufficiency either congenital or apoplectic, some forms of poisoning (see page 150) and in hot weather cystic fibrosis with heat stroke.

Treatment—see page 54.

ACUTE COLLAPSE IN INFANCY

Important Causes

Most commonly this is due to overwhelming infections such as gastro-enteritis or Gram-negative septicaemia, rarely hyponatraemia or adrenocortical crisis. A petechial rash would make the diagnosis of meningococcal septicaemia likely.

Initial clinical features may be minimal or may be those of rapid onset of profound shock, extreme pallor, cold extremities, mottled cyanosis, unobtainable blood pressure and acidotic respirations.

Immediate Resuscitation

Ensure a clear airway.

Commence intravenous therapy with either plasma, blood or dextran. If none of those is immediately available use 0·9 per cent saline. Rate: 20 ml/kg over 1 hour or less I.V.

If no improvement give hydrocortisone 100 mg intravenously. Treatment of severe disseminated intravascular coagulation (DIC) may also be considered.

Essential Investigations—having achieved an adequate circulation:

Full blood count and platelets—screening for DIC may be indicated. Blood urea, Dextrostix or blood glucose and electrolyte concentrations. Before antibiotic treatment is started investigations such as blood culture, lumbar puncture (warning, see page 125), rectal swab and throat swab must be carried out. Obtain urine specimen with the aid of a plastic bag; however do not delay treatment for this, but proceed to suprapubic aspiration of urine.

Further treatment will depend upon the findings *BUT:*

Ensure that a complete fluid balance chart is kept.

Anticipate the development of cerebral oedema (see p. 124).

D.C.A.C.

HYPONATRAEMIA AND ADRENOCORTICAL CRISIS

Hyponatraemia is usually due to haemodilution because of water retention (inappropriate ADH secretion) or inappropriate use of I.V. fluids. It can also be due to excessive salt loss in the urine, faeces, vomit or sweat. In the immature baby (<36 weeks gestation) the failure to reabsorb Na^+ in the renal tubules and an inadequate sodium intake from pooled expressed breast milk (EBM) are the most frequent causes. In the sick newborn or older child with diffuse pulmonary disease (e.g. bronchiolitis) or with cerebral oedema, inappropriate ADH production is the more likely diagnosis. Between one week and two months the salt-losing variety of congenital adrenal hyperplasia (CAH) (see below) heads the list. Once CAH is excluded renal failure and tubular acidosis (RTA) have to be considered. At any age Addison's disease and adrenocortical failure following prolonged systemic (sometimes topical) corticosteroid therapy (see below) or diuretic-induced renal sodium loss should not be forgotten.

Investigations

Take blood for Na, K, creatinine and urea and osmolality, pH and standard bicarbonate.

Collect random urine for Na, K, urea and creatine concentration, pH, osmolality and deposit. Start TIMED urine collections.

For interpretation of results see Fig. 3.

Principles of Management of Hyponatraemia

1. If haemodilution (incl. inappropriate ADH secretion) restrict fluids±diuretics.

2. For CAH or other causes of adrenocortical failure—see below.

3. For hyponatraemia in hypotonic dehydration—see page 54.

4. If hyponatraemia is due to diuretics, inappropriate I.V. fluids, vomiting, renal tubular loss, inadequate intake—correction with 0·9 per cent saline (or in certain cases more hypertonic saline) I.V. or addition of salt to diet as appropriate. May need to treat coexisting acidosis—page 57.

LOW SERUM SODIUM
↓
estimate serum K
↙ ⟶
if High   if Low
probable diagnoses   probable diagnoses

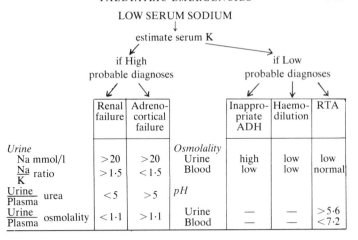

	Renal failure	Adreno-cortical failure		Inappropriate ADH	Haemo-dilution	RTA
Urine			*Osmolality*			
Na mmol/l	>20	>20	Urine	high	low	low
$\frac{Na}{K}$ ratio	>1.5	<1.5	Blood	low	low	normal
$\frac{Urine}{Plasma}$ urea	<5	>5	*pH*			
$\frac{Urine}{Plasma}$ osmolality	<1.1	>1.1	Urine	—	—	>5.6
			Blood	—	—	<7.2

FIG. 3.—Hyponatraemia: interpretation of results.

ADRENOCORTICAL FAILURE

(a) Following Long-term Corticosteroid Therapy

Children should be withdrawn gradually from treatment and it is reasonable to provide ACTH stimulation during the withdrawal period (40 i.u. twice weekly).

The pituitary-adrenal axis may remain depressed for as long as 2 years after steroid therapy over which period any operation or severe illness requires replacement therapy. (See page 267.)

(b) Salt-losing Syndrome and Congenital Adrenal Hyperplasia (CAH)

Babies suffering from CAH present with an adrenocortical crisis in the second or third week of life. The abnormal external genitalia and the determination of nuclear chromatin should provide an easy diagnosis in girls. The prompt diagnosis in boys is difficult (pigmented nipples and scrotum, low serum Na, high K with paradoxically high urine Na). Biochemical diagnosis in both sexes requires the determination of serum androgens and plasma 17-hydroxyprogesterone or if these are not available the determination of the 11-oxygenation index in the urine, the measurement of pregnanetriol and 17-oxosteroid excretion.

Treatment

Whatever the cause of the crisis treatment is urgent. It requires, at first, the rapid intravenous infusion of 0·9 per cent saline with glucose, together with hydrocortisone. Hydrocortisone 100 mg should be given intravenously at once and may be repeated at 2–6 hourly intervals depending on progress at all ages. Inadequate therapy is a common fault, both as regards sodium and hydrocortisone. Even babies may require 3 to 5 g of sodium chloride daily and a salt-retaining hormone should be given. Oral 9 alpha-fludrohydrocortisone 0·1 mg for a baby is appropriate, more for an older child. Hypoglycaemia (page 123) may remain unrecognised and untreated. Infusion therapy should be maintained for 1–2 days. Oedema and hypertension are the signs of excessive therapy.

Maintenance therapy should be trebled prophylactically if sufficient infection or stress occurs.

M.H.W.

HYPOGLYCAEMIA

Treat symptomatic hypoglycaemia by the prompt administration of intravenous dextrose after samples of blood have been taken for blood glucose (and if appropriate, insulin) levels (see page 198). An initial injection of 0·5 g/kg body weight given as 25 or 50 per cent solution should be followed by a continuous infusion of 5 or 10 per cent dextrose to deliver 5–10 mg/kg/min. If a rate greater than 15 mg/kg/min is required to prevent recurrence, hyperinsulinism should be suspected. The dextrose infusion should be withdrawn gradually to avoid rebound hypoglycaemia.

Long-term management.—Definitive treatment depends on the underlying cause. Glucocorticoids are specific for adrenal insufficiency but are usually ineffective in hypoglycaemia due to hyperinsulinism. The action of glucagon is transient and a longer-acting preparation has not been found useful. Diazoxide suppresses insulin secretion and may be valuable in hyperinsulinism given in a dose of 10–15 mg/kg/day in divided doses.

STATUS EPILEPTICUS

In this condition a succession of fits occurs without the patient recovering consciousness between them. It is a most serious state and, unless arrested, may leave permanent sequelae.

Emergency Treatment (for newborn see page 92)
1. Clear and maintain airway by suction and oropharyngeal airway: O_2 by face mask: be ready to intubate.
2. (*a*) Diazepam I.V. 0·3 mg/kg (I.M. unreliable). If vein inaccessible or if no response to I.V. injection in 10 minutes, give
   (*b*) Paraldehyde 0·1 ml/kg to 1 year, 1 ml/yr of age to 5 years+0·5 ml for each additional year to a maximum of 10 ml by deep I.M. injection—preferably 5 ml into each buttock. (Plastic syringes *may* be used *provided* paraldehyde is drawn up immediately before injection.) Although paraldehyde may be safely given again in 30 minutes, if fits do not rapidly come under control do not wait; go on to give:

(*c*) I.V. phenytoin (or phenobarbitone) 10 mg/kg; if that fails

(*d*) consider general anaesthesia and muscle relaxants.

3. As convulsions come under control:

Give phenobarbitone 6 mg/kg I.M. to a maximum of 90 mg below 12 years (unless phenytoin or phenobarbitone already used in 2*c*) to produce an extended anticonvulsant action, or

4. If I.V. diazepam initially effective and fits recur, use diazepam 50 micrograms/kg/h (dilute 40 mg in 500 ml 4 per cent dextrose/0·18 per cent saline or 5 per cent dextrose) by constant infusion.

Supportive Treatment

(*a*) Put up drip: very slow (1–2 ml/hour) infusion of 5 per cent dextrose or 4 per cent dextrose/0·18 per cent saline.

(*b*) Dextrostix for hypoglycaemia 3-hourly till recovery ensured.

(*c*) Record B.P. and temperature hourly.

(*d*) If temperature >40°C., tepid sponge, fan.

(*e*) Remember cerebral oedema may be playing a part after a prolonged fit. Treat with dexamethasone 0·1 mg/kg I.V. stat, then 0·05 mg/kg every 6 hours, and/or mannitol 20 per cent 7 ml/kg I.V. over 30 minutes after consultation.

(*f*) If progressive metabolic acidosis H^+ ion concentration >80 nmol/l (pH <7·1) treat cautiously as per page 57.

Causes

Consider intracranial vascular accident, other intracranial lesion, including abscess, meningo-encephalitis, hypertension and lead encephalopathy, acute porphyria, drugs, Reye's syndrome. (See investigations under Coma—below.) Hypoglycaemia, hypocalcaemia and hypomagnesaemia also need exclusion. Phenothiazines may cause oculogyric crises which may be misrepresented as fits.

COMA

First check position of patient, airway clear and ventilation satisfactory.

If preceding history uninformative, ask about drugs and

medication used in the home and get samples: also consider post-convulsive state (for causes, see above).

Examination for:

(1) Odour of breath, respiratory pattern, depth of coma, presence/absence of swallowing/coughing reflexes.

(2) Localising CNS signs. (3) Fundi: papilloedema/haemorrhages/vascular changes. (4) Neck stiffness. (5) B.P. (6) Signs of injury. (7) Skin rashes.

In the absence of history and localising signs, drug ingestion is most likely (especially up to 4 years).

Collect urine:

(a) for microscopy/protein/reducing substances/acetone, Phenistix (for aspirin);

(b) for ingested drugs—phone Poison Centre (page 149):

(c) for amino acids/porphobilinogen/porphyrins (for lead, page 158).

Collect blood for urea and creatinine, electrolytes, transaminases, glucose, Astrup, FBC and examination of film.

Lumbar puncture is indicated if meningitis or subarachnoid haemorrhage are suspected. If there is papilloedema or a suspicion of chronically raised pressure (**suggestive symptoms for more than three days**) contact neurosurgeon beforehand. The CSF pressure should always be measured and, if raised with a clear fluid, the neurosurgeon must be informed immediately so that steps to prevent the likely "cone" can be initiated forthwith.

X-rays: skull, chest, also bone ends (wrist and knee) and abdomen for signs of lead.

C.A.T. scan.

Causes are similar to those for Status Epilepticus (see page 124).

J.I.

HYDROCEPHALUS AND BLOCKED SHUNT

When the shunt becomes blocked, children may present with rapid and progressive rise in intracranial pressure leading to coma, blindness and respiratory arrest. Percutaneous needle aspiration of the reservoir, provided the ventricular catheter is patent, may be life-saving. The problem is less when the fontanelle is still open, in which case a lumbar puncture needle can be inserted into the ventricle through its lateral corner. When the ventricular catheter is occluded (shunt reservoir does not refill, needle aspiration unsuccessful) acute shunt malfunction is likely and requires urgent neurosurgical advice.

Blockage of the tube at cardiac or peritoneal end often produces less dramatic symptoms and signs. Signs of raised intracranial pressure may be absent but unexplained anorexia, vomiting, apathy and failure to thrive pervade. Valves may become infected, usually with *Staph. albus* (alias micrococcus). There may be fever, positive blood culture or culture from valve, but some cases present with microscopic haematuria and progressive renal failure from shunt nephritis. Persistent infection may be confirmed by the detection of raised antibodies to the organism.

A.D.H.

RESPIRATORY EMERGENCIES

1. Upper Airway Obstruction

Presents with stridor due to such causes as epiglottitis, laryngotracheobronchitis, foreign body, angioneurotic oedema and very rarely diphtheria. Causes of persistent stridor in the neonate include congenital laryngeal stridor (infantile larynx), sub-glottic haemangioma, vocal cord palsy, laryngeal webs, cysts, papillomata and subglottic stenosis.

Epiglottitis should be distinguished from the other causes by its rapid onset over a few hours, associated with a high temperature and a severely ill child. It is associated with a septicaemia due to group B *Haemophilus influenzae*. The patient has difficulty in swallowing and oral feeds are contra-indicated. Inspection of the throat may precipitate a respiratory arrest and should only be performed with an anaesthetist at hand. Do not sedate. Take blood cultures, and treat with chloramphenicol and intravenous fluids. Intubation is indicated in all patients unless constantly observed by an anaesthetist. If facilities for the nursing of patients with nasotracheal tubes are inadequate, tracheostomy is indicated. Both nasal and tracheostomy tubes must be adequately humidified.

2. Lower Airway Obstruction

Presents with expiratory wheeze. Causes include asthma, bronchiolitis (see below), foreign body, cystic fibrosis and more rarely tuberculous lymph glands and tracheal abnormalities.

3. Other Causes of Respiratory Difficulty

(*a*) *Pulmonary* causes include pneumonia, lobar emphysema, pneumothorax, mediastinal emphysema.

(*b*) *Cardiac.*—Heart failure can easily be missed and is sometimes precipitated and masked by an infection. The heart rate and the size of the liver are important guides (see page 142).

(*c*) *Metabolic acidosis.*—Deep, sighing respirations should raise the possibility of diabetes mellitus (smell of acetone), aspirin poisoning, "uraemia", periodic syndrome or fulminating infections such as meningococcal septicaemia or gastro-enteritis. Check Astrup values and test urine with Acetest.

ACUTE BRONCHIOLITIS

This condition is often preceded by coryza followed by increasing dyspnoea, paroxysmal cough and failure to feed. Clinical signs in the chest may be minimal but generalised inspiratory crepitations, emphysema and expiratory wheeze are often found. The chest X-ray shows emphysema only, unless secondary atelectasis or pneumonia has occurred.

Treatment

Oxygen.

Maintain airway free from excess secretions by suction.

Maintain hydration, if necessary by tube feeding. Intravenous fluids are needed if vomiting occurs, if gastric distension hinders respiration and in sick infants.

Broad-spectrum antibiotics only if secondary bacterial invasion is suspected.

Undue restlessness is likely to be due to hypoxia or CO_2 retention. Blood gases should be monitored. Sedation is contra-indicated.

Heart failure is a very rare complication, usually only occurring in babies with congenital heart disease.

If clinical condition is deteriorating and Pco_2 rising, endotracheal intubation and assisted ventilation should be considered.

STATUS ASTHMATICUS

Status asthmaticus in infants and young children produces an increase in the work of respiration, arterial hypoxaemia and metabolic and respiratory acidosis. Baseline values of acid base balance and Po_2 should be obtained if available.

Immediate Treatment

DO NOT give loading doses of aminophylline to any child on chronic oral theophylline treatment. Avoid sedation or aminophylline suppositories.

Give:
1. Oxygen.
2. Nebulised sympathomimetic, e.g. salbutamol or terbutaline respirator solution (0·25 ml–1·5 ml respirator solution according to age of child, diluted in 0·9 per cent saline to give a total volume of 2–3 ml) via a nebuliser driven by oxygen or air from a compressor;
OR, if not available, salbutamol I.V. 5 micrograms/kg over 10 minutes.
3. Aminophylline I.V. 4 mg/kg over 20 minutes.

Follow-up Treatment

If child has not substantially improved on above treatment set up I.V. drip of 4 per cent dextrose in 0·18 per cent saline, if not already started, and continue at rate of 70–120 ml/kg/day.

Give: Hydrocortisone I.V. 4 mg/kg/2-hourly, reducing to 2 mg/kg/2-hourly when response occurs and

Aminophylline I.V. 0·7 mg/kg/h., together with nebulised salbutamol or terbutaline as above 4-hourly.

X-ray chest to exclude pneumothorax or pneumonia; antibiotics need not be given unless infection is likely. Monitor blood gases in severe cases and peak expiratory flow rate in co-operative patients.

Later Treatment

As soon as the child can take by mouth, start:

Oral prednisolone 0·5 mg/kg/6-hourly, and continue nebulised salbutamol or terbutaline if possible. Oral bronchodilators may have to be substituted in younger patients.

Prednisolone should be continued until improvement has occurred and then discontinued over 3–5 days. Previous outpatient treatment should be reviewed and modified before discharge.

SIGNS OF RESPIRATORY FAILURE

These are indicated by:

1. Decreasing respiratory effort from exhaustion and, despite severe airways obstruction, decreased expiratory wheeze.

2. Impaired consciousness.

3. Persistent cyanosis despite adequate oxygen therapy.

4. Increasing respiratory acidosis with P_{CO_2} in excess of 8 kPa.

If these signs persist despite adequate drug therapy, mechanically assisted ventilation in an intensive therapy unit will be indicated.

P.H.W.

ACUTE RENAL PROBLEMS

NEPHROTIC SYNDROME

More than 80 per cent of children with the nephrotic syndrome respond to corticosteroid therapy in adequate dosage, e.g. prednisone 60 mg/m^2/day, which should be continued until the urine has been protein-free (Albustix negative or trace) for three consecutive days, and then tapered until discontinued within 1–2 weeks. Three types of emergency may arise in a nephrotic child.

1. Hypovolaemia

This results from plasma albumin depletion and is partly compensated by sodium and water retention, through activation of the renin-aldosterone system. When serum albumin levels fall below about 15 g/l, hypovolaemia may have significant consequences. The main clinical features consist of abdominal pain, tachycardia and cold extremities. The GFR falls and, in extreme cases, particularly where frusemide has been given in excess and has exacerbated the hypovolaemia, acute renal failure may develop.

The aim of management should be to recognise impending severe hypovolaemia and prevent deterioration. Salt-poor albumin should be infused intravenously, a dose of 0·5 g/kg being given over a period of 2–3 h when the serum albumin is 10–15 g/l, and 1·0 g/kg when it is below 10 g/l. Frusemide should be given simultaneously, a bolus of 2 mg/kg being injected into the drip about half an hour after starting. Too rapid an infusion of albumin carries a potentially fatal hazard of vascular overload, with pulmonary oedema, and combination with frusemide diminishes this risk. Both lead through different mechanisms to salt and water diuresis, with benefit to the patient. The effect is transient owing to continuing proteinuria, but the schedule may be repeated at 6-hourly intervals, as required.

If the child is already in a state of severe oliguria with azotaemia, conservative treatment for acute renal failure (p. 132) must be instituted, proceeding if necessary to peritoneal dialysis.

2. Peritonitis

The urinary losses of IgG together with the presence of ascitic fluid increases the vulnerability of the peritoneum to bacterial infection. The differential diagnosis may present difficulty particularly in the patient who is already receiving corticosteroids, which may mask the signs of peritonism. The possibility of acute appendicitis should be considered and may call for experienced surgical opinion. Remember that hypovolaemia may present with acute abdominal pain, while steroids may induce a misleading leucocytosis. Needling the peritoneal cavity for culture is generally unrewarding and it is safer to assume the presence of infection if in doubt and treat it vigorously with broad-spectrum antibiotics, bearing in mind that either pneumococci or Gram-negative organisms may cause it.

3. Chickenpox and Measles

The parents of the nephrotic child who is non-immune to these infections must be warned of their potential dangers if contracted during steroid therapy. Close contact with varicella—e.g. in the home or school class—should be notified immediately and zoster immune globulin injected intramuscularly within 48 h. Fortunately most children will already have received live measles vaccine and will be at least partially protected. While during the pre-steroid era measles was sometimes observed to induce a nephrotic remission, both infections, and particularly varicella, may also provoke a relapse. In this case, the child should be nursed at home or, if necessary, admitted into isolation, for observation and diuretic therapy if oedematous. Prednisone should be withheld until the signs of viraemia are receding, since remission may then occur spontaneously, making treatment unnecessary. If not done already, measles vaccination should be performed during remission, not less than a month after cessation of steroid therapy.

ACUTE RENAL FAILURE

Acute renal failure usually presents with severe oliguria but is occasionally diagnosed in the presence of a normal urine output, especially when caused by severe burns. It may occur as a complication of four main conditions:

1. Hypovolaemia or hypotension, as in blood loss, dehydration, septicaemia, burns, major cardiac surgery, and the nephrotic syndrome.
2. Renal tubular poisoning.
3. Glomerular disease as in glomerulonephritis or the haemolytic-uraemic syndrome.
4. Bilateral renal vein thrombosis, mainly in dehydrated infants.

Most causes are potentially reversible and all types should be treated energetically with recovery in view.

Three phases are recognisable: (i) Potentially reversible oliguria (pre-renal failure); (ii) established renal failure; (iii) diuretic phase.

Treatment depends on the stage in which the patient is first seen. In all cases urinary obstruction (e.g. posterior urethral valves in boys, faecal impaction in girls) should first be ruled out by palpation or ultrasonic scan of the bladder.

Catheterisation is generally necessary initially, for diagnostic purposes, but an in-dwelling catheter should be avoided because of the risk of infection. Renal size should be assessed ultrasonically and a plain radiograph taken to exclude opaque calculi.

The following data should be obtained immediately: (i) body weight; (ii) serum electrolytes, osmolality, urea, creatinine, calcium, acid-base status, haemoglobin, haematocrit and blood for group and cross-match; (iii) urinary osmolality and urea.

1. Potentially Reversible Oliguria

Treat vigorously to remove underlying cause, i.e. hypovolaemia, dehydration or obstruction. Dehydration should be assessed (see p. 53) and corrected as rapidly as possible with an isotonic fluid. If the random urine:plasma (U:P) urea ratio is 5 or more and the U:P osmolality ratio 1·1 or more, the oliguria is physiological and should respond to rehydration. If oliguria (<200 ml/24 hours/m²) persists after rehydration and the U:P urea and osmolality ratios are low, the patient should be given mannitol 0·75 g/kg (e.g. 3·5 ml/kg of a 20 per cent solution) intravenously in 5 minutes followed if necessary by frusemide 5 mg/kg intravenously 15 minutes later. Alternatively, proceed straight to intravenous frusemide, omitting the mannitol. If there is still no diuresis, confirmed if necessary by bladder catheterisation, management for established renal failure must be started *immediately* to prevent fluid overload.

Pre-renal oliguria due to the nephrotic syndrome requires completely different management, as described on page 131.

2. Established Renal Failure

Successful management demands careful attention to the following:

(a) Fluid requirements

Overhydration may have occurred during the early phase of treatment, causing plasma dilution with reduced sodium levels; the temptation to correct this with sodium supplements must be resisted.

The daily fluid requirement is the sum of:

(i) Extrarenal insensible loss less water derived from metabolic processes. Allow 15 ml/kg in infants, 12 ml/kg in older children. This value should be increased by 10 per cent for each 1°C fever present.

(ii) Gastro-intestinal losses.

(iii) Urine output. In practice the preceding day's urine output is used. Fluid balance should be recorded as accurately as possible but frequent weighing is the only reliable guide. With proper management, tissue break-down will cause a daily weight loss of the order of 0·5 per cent of body weight.

(b) Electrolyte requirements

Sodium: No significant urinary loss will occur during oliguria. Gastro-intestinal losses, i.e. diarrhoea and vomiting, must be replaced by a fluid of similar electrolyte composition (see page 58).

Potassium: A steady rise in the serum level occurs from protein catabolism and cellular disruption. No additional potassium should be given during the oliguric phase. The ECG provides a valuable guide to impending toxicity. For emergency treatment of cardiotoxic effects, correct acidosis and give (i) I.V. glucose 4 g/kg with 1 unit soluble insulin/4 g glucose; (ii) calcium gluconate 10 per cent, 0·3 ml/kg; (iii) Resonium A 0·5 g/kg orally or rectally. These will control the hyperkalaemia for 3–4 hours until dialysis can be arranged.

(c) *Calorie and protein requirement:*

Both are necessary to reduce catabolism and delay azot-aemia and hyperkalaemia. 50–100 cals/kg/day should be given mainly as concentrated carbohydrate (Hycal and Caloreen by mouth) and fat (intravenous preparations or oral Prosparol). The limiting factors are volume and palatability. High-class protein, e.g. egg or low-sodium milks, should also be given in amounts ranging from 0·5 g/kg/day (older children) to 1·5 g/kg/day (infants).

(d) *Drugs*

Prophylactic antibiotics are not indicated. Many drugs are excreted largely by the kidney and dosage should be controlled by measurement of blood levels. When this is not possible, normal doses should be given at increased intervals which are determined by the metabolism and routes of excretion of each drug.

Indications for dialysis

If oliguria is prolonged or the child is intensely hypercata-bolic, as in massive burns or septicaemia, clinical and meta-bolic deterioration may occur despite careful conservative management, and dialysis is required. The indications vary in individual patients and the following is only an approximate guide:

Serum potassium greater than 7 mmol/l, or ECG changes.

Blood urea greater than 40 mmol/l (240 mg/100 ml).

Plasma bicarbonate less than 13 mmol/l.

Uncontrolled hypertension.

Overhydration—oedema and weight gain.

Progressive clinical deterioration, e.g. drowsiness, convul-sions.

Peritoneal dialysis is generally used but, in certain instances, e.g. peritonitis, abdominal wall burns, haemodialysis is indi-cated. The former is comparatively simple and cheap, but is undoubtedly safer and more effective in the hands of larger paediatric units with special facilities for treatment and monitoring.

3. **Diuretic Phase**

Sodium, potassium and water depletion may occur at this

stage, owing to faulty tubular reabsorption, but can generally be corrected orally.

Hypertensive Crises

Severe hypertension may be caused by sodium overload or by renin/angiotensin excess in both acute and chronic renal failure and in other forms of renal disease (e.g. reflux nephropathy) without failure. For encephalopathy or when the diastolic B.P. is over 120 mm Hg, intravenous diazoxide 5 mg/kg should be used and repeated as necessary. Where vascular overload is a major factor, frusemide (2·0 mg/kg) should also be given intravenously. Stabilisation with oral therapy should be initiated as soon as possible, using propranolol unless contra-indicated, combined with hydralazine. Once intravenous diazoxide and frusemide have been discontinued, bendrofluazide should be added, and as the blood pressure becomes controlled it may be possible to reduce and discontinue the hydralazine. If oral therapy is not possible initially, hydralazine can be given parenterally (0·2 mg/kg/dose).

R.H.R.W.

DIABETES MELLITUS
Treatment of Diabetic Ketoacidosis

This regime should be used in newly presenting or established diabetic children if any of the following signs are present:

Significant dehydration, vomiting, acidotic respiration, heavy ketonuria, impaired level of consciousness (provided hypoglycaemia has been excluded).

Initial investigations.—Blood glucose, Astrup values, electrolytes and infection screen.

Treatment need not await results. Record body weight and chart fluid input and output accurately.

Initial Management

Fluids: Give nil by mouth; assume 10 per cent dehydration + basic maintenance and use 0·9 per cent saline as initial infusion, calculating amount from the following table:

Age yrs	Weight kg	Rehydration ml	+	Maintenance ml/kg	or	Maintenance total ml	=	Total Vol/ 24 h as ml
1	10	1000		120		1200		2200
5	18	1800		100		1800		3600
10	30	3000		75		2250		5250
15	50	5000		50		2500		7500

Give ⅓ of 24 h requirement in first 4 hours
Give ⅓ of 24 h requirement in next 8 hours
Give ⅓ of 24 h requirement in next 12 hours

These are *maximal* volumes. If severe hyperosmolality is present [2 (Na+K)+glucose+urea] = >340 mosmol, reduce initial fluid to 75 per cent of requirements, or to 50 per cent of requirements if osmolality >400 mosmol. Change to 4·3 per cent dextrose 0·18 per cent saline when blood glucose < 15·0 mmol/l. Reduce I.V. fluids accordingly when oral fluids are commenced.

Subsequent investigations.—Repeat blood glucose, electrolytes and acid base balance at 2–4-hourly intervals until blood glucose is less than 15 mmol/l.

Subsequent Management

Oral feeding can usually begin about 12 hours after

admission with small (15–30 ml) quantities hourly. Fluids should include glucose 20 g 3-hourly and potassium supplements or fruit juices.

Further subcutaneous soluble insulin should be given according to the blood sugar level or amount of glycosuria and ketonuria.

Urine glucose g/100 ml	Ketonuria present or absent	Blood glucose mmol/l	Insulin units/kg
5	+	20 or +	0·5
5 2	0 } +	15–20	0·4
2 1	0 } +	10–15	0·3
1	–	5–10	0·2
0–0·5	–	5 or –	0·1

Insulin

Use soluble insulin, e.g. Actrapid MC (Novo), Velosulin (Nordisk), Neusulin (Wellcome). Give 0·05 unit/kg/body weight I.M. stat. followed by 0·05 unit/kg/body weight every hour until the blood glucose is less than 15 mmol/l (270 mg/100 ml). The rate of fall of blood glucose should not exceed 4–5 mmol/h because of the danger of cerebral oedema which may follow a rapid reduction in blood osmolality. Remember that established diabetics may have a depot of subcutaneous insulin which will be absorbed as the circulation improves.

Alternatively 0·1 unit/kg of soluble insulin may be given intravenously stat. followed by the continuous I.V. infusion of the same body weight dose hourly, using an infusion pump. The larger dosage is required to compensate for absorption of insulin onto the surface of the infusion tubing.

Potassium

Await serum potassium values and ensure urine output. If initial level is less than 5·0 mmol/l give 6 mmol/kg/day as potassium chloride intravenously but do not exceed an infusion concentration of greater than 30 mmol/l. An ECG monitor to observe T wave changes is helpful.

Bicarbonate

The metabolic acidosis will resolve without specific correction in all but the most severe cases.

If (H^+) concentration is less than 80 nmol/l (pH >7·1) no bicarbonate is necessary.

If (H^+) concentration is 80–100 nmol/l (pH 7·1–7·0) give 0·5 mmol/kg $NaHCO_3$ over 15 minutes I.V.

If (H^+) concentration exceeds 100 nmol/l (pH <7·0) give 0·75 mmol/kg/$NaHCO_3$ over 15 minutes I.V.

Insulin doses may initially be given 4-hourly, followed by six-hourly and then three times daily before meals when the patient has commenced a light diet.

WITHOUT SEVERE ACIDOSIS OR DEHYDRATION

Most children are in this group at the time of diagnosis and stabilisation can usually be achieved by the following regime:

Insulin

Soluble insulin in a dose of approximately 0·5 units/kg is given subcutaneously three times daily at the start of each main meal according to the above scheme. Some insulin will be necessary when urine tests are negative. Parental education in diabetic management should begin at this stage.

When ketonuria has disappeared and moderate stabilisation has been achieved, a change to a once- or twice-daily insulin routine may be made, using initially about ¾ of the total daily soluble dose. In general, very young children (0–3 yr) are best controlled on twice-daily soluble insulin, children 3–10 years by a medium or longer-acting insulin such as Monotard MC (Novo) and older children (11–16 yr) by a twice-daily soluble and isophane mixture such as Velosulin and Insulatard (Nordisk).

Diet

The daily calories are apportioned approximately as follows: Carbohydrate 40–45 per cent, protein 15–20 per cent, fat 35–40 per cent. The carbohydrate intake is regulated through the day, the basis for the calculation being the quantity of each item of food which contains 10 g of carbohydrate (= 1 portion = 40 kcal). The total daily portions of carbohydrate are divided into roughly equal amounts for breakfast, lunch and supper with "snacks" of roughly 10–20 g (1–2 portions) for mid-morning and 30–40 g (3–4 portions) at tea-time.

About 1,000 kilocalories per day are necessary at one year, increasing by approximately 100 kilocalories per day for each year of age until puberty. The calorie content of the diet should be decided before discharge but final stabilisation of insulin dosage is only possible at home. There may be value in increasing the amount of roughage in the diet by incorporating bran, beans and unrefined carbohydrate such as wholemeal bread.

P.H.W.R.

CONGENITAL HEART LESIONS AND CARDIAC EMERGENCIES

Newborn babies going into heart failure or showing progressive cyanosis need urgent investigation. Once symptoms develop deterioration is often rapid and a few hours' delay may prove fatal. Immediate referral to a paediatric cardiology centre is advised as open heart surgery, when necessary, is now possible at any age or weight.

Acyanotic conditions liable to cause signs of heart failure and respiratory distress in the newborn period include obstructive lesions of the left heart such as the coarctation syndrome (coarctation±other cardiac lesion) and hypoplastic left heart syndrome. In infancy coarctation of the aorta and L→R shunts are the most common causes. The more severe newborn lesions may lead to massive liver enlargement and intense metabolic acidosis.

Cyanotic congenital heart conditions commonly include transposition of the great arteries, severe Fallot's tetralogy and tricuspid atresia.

Dysrhythmias.—Paroxysmal tachycardia is the commonest dysrhythmia in infants. Diagnosis must be made on ECG. The heart rate is rapid and regular. Digoxin is usually effective but it might render later DC countershock hazardous. Initial treatment may include the cautious, slow intravenous injection of verapamil*, under careful ECG and blood pressure monitoring. The "cardiac arrest" team should be standing by. *Propranolol should never be used in conjunction with verapamil, and vice versa.*

Ventricular arrhythmias are uncommon and can be recognised only by electrocardiography. They are treated by intravenous mexiletine*, lignocaine* or procainamide*.

Congenital heart block can occur without other cardiac abnormality or may be associated with corrected transposition, or myocarditis. The condition rarely requires treatment but a persistently slow pulse rate (usually less than 40 per minute) may cause heart failure or syncopal attacks and should then be treated by intravenous isoprenaline (2–4 mg in 500 ml of 50 g/l dextrose) infused fast enough to increase the rate to about 80 per minute, until cardiac pacing by intravenous electrode can be used.

* See literature for dosage.

Heart Failure

The usual symptoms in infancy are breathlessness, slow feeding and inability to complete feeds. The heart is enlarged (best seen on X-ray) and there is dyspnoea, hepatomegaly and tachycardia. There may be unexplained or disproportionate weight gain due to fluid retention.

Management

Commence treatment for heart failure and then consider referral to a paediatric cardiology unit.

Initially the following measures may be tried:

1. Frusemide in adequate doses (start with 1–2 mg/kg I.M. or 1 mg/kg I.V.; if diuresis not produced within 2 hours a repeat single dose of up to 4 mg/kg I.M. may be tried)—for usual maintenance dose see page 239.
2. Oxygen.
3. Tube-feeding.
4. Digoxin—use maintenance dose 5 micrograms/kg twice daily (see p. 238).
5. Potassium supplement.
6. Semi-upright position.

Cyanotic Attacks

These attacks are particularly common in children with Fallot's tetralogy. They are characterised by rapid appearance of severe cyanosis, breathlessness and occasional loss of consciousness. The systolic murmur becomes fainter and shorter and may disappear. The child should be nursed in the knee/elbow position and given oxygen. Intravenous propranolol should be given at a rate of 0·1 mg/kg/min, the total dose not to exceed 0·5–1·0 mg/kg. (See p. 244.) The drug should be stopped if there is a significant fall in blood pressure or pulse rate. It is important to avoid dehydration in all types of cyanotic heart disease because of the danger of vascular thrombosis, particularly during intercurrent infection.

Antibiotics

Antibiotic cover must be given to all children with congenital and rheumatic heart disease if teeth are to be extracted or an operation is undertaken: the traditional treatment is to give 300,000 units of procaine penicillin I.M. at the time, followed by oral penicillin, 250 mg four times daily for one week, but the initial and crucial injection is often missed out. The alternative is to give a single dose of amoxycillin by mouth 2 hours before dental treatment as follows: 1–7 yr, 750 mg; 7–14 yr, 1·5 g; 14 yr+, 3 g. If the child is on prophylactic penicillin and a tooth has to be extracted a different antiobiotic should be given.

Children with rheumatic heart disease need continuous penicillin prophylaxis to reduce the likelihood of relapse (penicillin V, 125 mg twice daily).

CARDIORESPIRATORY ARREST

The commonest cause of a "cardiac arrest call" is a respiratory arrest with a secondary cardiac arrest. Causes include inhalation of vomit, anoxia, anaesthetics and other drugs, hyperkalaemia, and as a result of serious arrhythmias during cardiac catheterisation.

Immediate action

Summon emergency team, clear airway and maintain ventilation by mouth-to-mouth respiration or endotracheal intubation until anaesthetist arrives. Start external cardiac massage: place child on firm surface, compress sternum with heel of hand, rhythmically 60 times per minute*. Success judged by feeling temporal pulse. Aspirate pharynx intermittently and continue until emergency team arrives.

Emergency Team

Anaesthetist is usually responsible for ventilation, while another doctor should continue cardiac massage. Give sodium bicarbonate I.V. Assume base deficit of 20 mmol in infants, 30–40 mmol in older children. After Astrup determination, if metabolic acidosis persists give further bicarbonate according to formula on page 57.

Cardioversion.—Connect machine to mains and leads to patient. Record ECG on oscilloscope. If asystole is confirmed (straight line of oscilloscope) try to induce ventricular fibrillation by giving 2–3 ml of 1:10,000 solution of adrenaline and calcium gluconate 2–3 ml of 100 g/l solution or calcium chloride 100–200 mg intravenously or into the heart. For ventricular fibrillation use external DC countershock, 25–50

* 1 breath/4 chest compressions.

Joules initially for small infants, 75–200 Joules for older children, depending on size and age. Drugs should not be given into the heart if the patient is on positive pressure ventilation as this may precipitate a pneumothorax. Failure to restore sinus rhythm after defibrillation may be due to anoxia (check ventilation), metabolic acidosis (corrected by more bicarbonate) or a very irritable myocardium (tall, coarse ventricular fibrillatory waves on the oscilloscope) or insufficient Joules (use higher energy). In resistant cases of coarse ventricular fibrillation use lignocaine 10 mg or propranolol 1 mg or phenytoin sodium 5–10 mg intravenously or into the heart before attempting further DC shock with higher energy. If fine ventricular fibrillation persists with low voltage fibrillatory waves on ECG give adrenaline or calcium chloride before attempting further defibrillation. In some cases of asystole or resistant ventricular fibrillation transvenous pacing may be needed.

Resuscitation should be continued for as long as the patient responds or ECG evidence of cardiac depolarisation persists. (Dilated unresponsive pupils or flat EEG are ominous signs.)

Ventricular arrhythmias are common after resuscitation and are usually due to metabolic acidosis, anoxaemia or digoxin.

Treatment consists of correcting the acidosis and using a suitable anti-arrhythmic agent such as lignocaine, procainamide or a beta-blocking agent such as mexiletine. (See p. 141.) For management of post anoxic cerebral oedema see page 124.

E.D.S.

EXTENSIVE BURNS

Anoxia is the first complication to consider, especially if the face has been burned or the child has been in smoke. Causes are laryngeal obstruction, pulmonary oedema, contracted burned skin encircling the chest, carboxyhaemoglobin, anaemia and shock. If oxygen and humidification are not adequate, positive pressure ventilation will be needed.

If possible weigh the patient before treatment is started. Sedation is not indicated unless the child complains of continuing pain: papaveretum (see page 242) or diamorphine (0·1 mg/kg) can be given intravenously. Prescribe tetanus toxoid (0·5 ml I.M.) to the actively immunised; a 7-day course of systemic erythromycin estolate or flucloxacillin to the unprotected; and human anti-tetanus globulin, A.T.G., Humotet (Wellcome) 1 ml I.M. if treatment has been delayed, or the wound is heavily contaminated with soil or faeces. A urethral catheter should be passed if the burn is over 25 per cent.

If the burn extends over more than 10 per cent of the body surface, excluding erythema (i.e. one whole upper limb), the child will need intravenous therapy to prevent or correct shock. Colloid (plasma, plasma protein fraction, or dextran 110 in saline) is better than electrolyte solution alone but they can be given in equal proportions. Plasma equal to the child's plasma volume (see page 169) should be given for every 15 per cent of skin burned, one-half in the first 8 hours, and the other half in the next 16 hours. This rate should be adjusted to keep the capillary haematocrit near normal and the urine output at 1 ml/kg/hour. Water by mouth should be limited to three-quarters of the normal intake (see page 53). Blood is rarely needed in the shock stage but can be given at the end of it (usually an amount equal to 20–40 per cent of the blood volume for burns over 40 per cent). During the shock stage one should look for evidence of renal failure, which may be oliguric or non-oliguric.

If parts of the burn are deep, a surgeon should see the case early with a view to excision and skin grafting on the third or fourth days. (Analgesia to pin-prick signifies a deep dermal burn or full thickness skin destruction).

Feeding may be commenced, by nasogastric tube if necessary, 24 hours after burning. If oral feeding is not accepted, potassium should be given without further delay by mouth or intravenously in a generous amount to prevent ileus (see page 56).

The burn is a fistula leaking water, sodium and potassium. The rate of water loss through it averages 0·30 ml/cm² burned area/day. The average sodium loss is 0·03 mmol/cm² burned area/day. The protein loss is similar to dilute plasma, about 30 g/l. Extensively burned patients probably need 1½ times the calories and 2–3 times the protein needed in health and this should be achieved over several days.

D.McG.J.

VII

ACCIDENTAL POISONING

POISON INFORMATION CENTRES IN U.K.

(24-hour service providing detailed advice)

Telephone Numbers:

London 01-407 7600	Leeds 0532-32799
Cardiff 0222-492233	Belfast 0232–30503
Manchester 061–740 2254	Edinburgh 031-229 2477

The usual age group is 1–4 years with the maximum incidence around 2. Boys outnumber girls 2:1. Drugs account for the majority of cases, the remainder are mainly household substances.

INITIAL MANAGEMENT

Measures which are relevant to the treatment of all poisoned patients are the maintenance of an adequate airway, the removal and identification of the ingested substance and the management of any complications (supportive treatment). Whatever treatment is given should be carried out calmly and methodically—the indiscriminate use of antidotes, sedatives or stimulants can be more dangerous than the poison. *Milk* is very useful as a bland, soothing, buffering agent which can be given immediately. Specific antidotes are mentioned in the appropriate sections. Spillage on to the skin and into the eyes may be present and require attention. Children who are not admitted following ingestion should be observed for up to 4 hours in the Emergency Department before being allowed home.

Removal of the Ingested Poison

Stomach emptying is best achieved by vomiting; however, emesis should not be induced in the unconscious patient or after ingestion of corrosives (phenols, acids and caustic alkalis), paraffin (kerosene) or white spirit.

Methods

Immediate—push a spoon handle down the throat, easier if preceded by a drink of water or milk.

Emetic.—Ipecacuanha   Paediatric   Emetic   Draught

149

10–15 ml followed by 300–500 ml squash. The dose can be repeated once after 30 minutes if vomiting has not occurred. It may be ineffective after the ingestion of antiemetics, phenothiazines, atropine and amphetamines. Salt water should NEVER be used as an emetic (fatal consequences have been reported).

Gastric lavage should be used if removal is urgent. It should never be attempted on the unconscious patient without prior insertion of a cuffed endotracheal tube. It is not recommended after ingestion of paraffin (aspiration, lipoid pneumonia), or corrosives (perforation).

Method: wrap the child in a restraining sheet and lay on the left side. Tilt the table head down. Choose a tube with a large lumen (at least 28 F.G., 17 E.G.) and mark the distance from the bridge of the nose to the xiphisternum. Lubricate with water-soluble jelly. Pass by mouth to the mark using a padded mouth-peg between the teeth (check first for loose teeth). Make sure the tube is not in the trachea (coughing, continuous bubbling) and always aspirate for stomach contents before starting lavage. Lavage with 150–200 ml amounts of warm isotonic saline, 1 per cent sodium bicarbonate or tap water (note risk of water intoxication) and continue until the returned fluid is clear. A petechial rash often appears immediately after lavage, in the orbits and around hairline and neck. It fades after 24 hours.

Purges and enemata may remove unabsorbed material from the gut but can add to the irritant effect of the poison. A solution of sodium sulphate 300 mg/kg is recommended orally.

Activated charcoal can be left in the stomach after lavage or introduced by nasogastric tube. However, it inhibits the action of ipecacuanha so await vomiting before using it.

Osmotic diuresis with mannitol 3·5 ml/kg of a 20 per cent solution I.V. or hypertonic solutions of urea or dextrose will increase excretion of various poisons but may cause dangerous hypokalaemia if potassium-containing fluids are not administered. The excretion of salicylates and barbiturates is enhanced when osmotic diuresis is combined with an alkaline urine. Amphetamine excretion is enhanced in an acid urine.

Exchange transfusions have been used in poisoning by salicylates, iron, chlorinated hydrocarbons and copper sulphate.

Peritoneal dialysis and haemodialysis may be of value if the poison is diffusible and the toxicity is related to the blood concentration, e.g. barbiturates, salicylates. Indications are deep coma, apnoeic episodes, hypotension and oliguria.

Identification

The container and label should be obtained if possible but are not an absolute guide to identity of contents as these are sometimes transferred from one container to another. Tablets should be checked for colour, size and code against charts, e.g. Data Sheet Compendium. The prescriber, dispensing chemist, manufacturer or Poison Information Centre can provide information. These procedures are far quicker than analysis of specimens. Save (in order of usefulness) specimens of:

Vomitus or first gastric aspirate.

Urine—particularly if some hours after ingestion.

Venous blood.

Supportive Treatment

Recordings of temperature, pulse, respiration, blood pressure and fluid intake/output should be routine.

Temperature regulation.—Hyperpyrexia (over 40°C) should be treated by exposure, tepid water sponging and fans.

Hypothermia—cover with warmed blankets. The use of heat lamps, hot water bottles and pads can be dangerous if the patient is unconscious.

Pain should be adequately treated with analgesics.

Delirium and excitation. Chlorpromazine I.M. is recommended.

Antibiotics should be used to treat specific infections only.

Other measures are dealt with in the following sections: circulatory failure (page 119), respiratory failure (page 129), fluid and electrolyte balance (page 53), acidosis (page 57), convulsions and coma (page 123), nutrition (page 26), hypoglycaemia (page 123) and acute renal failure (page 132).

SPECIFIC POISONS

Salicylates

Peak blood levels may be reached between 2 and 3 hours[*]

[*] If enteric-coated observe in hospital for 24 hours.

after ingestion. Fifty per cent of ingested aspirin is excreted in the first 24 hours. 150–200 mg/kg of aspirin will cause symptoms.

Symptoms.—Initial hyperventilation produces respiratory alkalosis and renal compensation increases the urinary loss of base. This phase is usually short in children and is followed by metabolic acidosis. Carbohydrate metabolism is disturbed, causing ketosis but rarely hypoglycaemia. Dehydration, hyperpyrexia and hypoprothrombinaemia may also occur.

Investigations.—Serum salicylate—a level below 2·92 mmol/l (40 mg/100 ml) rarely causes symptoms, over 8·76 mmol/l (120 mg/100 ml) is usually lethal.

Blood H^+ concentration, Pco_2, standard bicarbonate, electrolytes, blood sugar and prothrombin time.

Urine gives a mauve to violet colour with Phenistix and violet with $FeCl_3$ persisting after boiling.

Treatment.—Emesis or gastric lavage with 1 per cent sodium bicarbonate even *up to 24 hours* after ingestion. Activated charcoal should be left in stomach.

Press oral fluids. Dextrose saline should be given I.V. if the child is vomiting or collapsed (100–150 ml/kg/24 hours).

Bicarbonate corrects the metabolic acidosis (page 57). It should not be given intravenously without estimating blood H^+ concentration. Alkalinising the urine increases the excretion of salicylate (2 mmol bicarbonate/kg should normally raise urine pH to 7 or more). In severe ketoacidosis bicarbonate may cause hypernatraemia; additional potassium should be given, provided renal function is adequate.

Acetazolamide 5 mg/kg given orally or I.M. 6–8-hourly also increases urinary salicylate excretion.

Hypoprothrombinaemia may be corrected by vitamin K_1 I.M. or I.V. and by transfusions.

Avoid giving CNS depressants, e.g. barbiturates, morphine.

Alkaline osmotic diuresis, dialysis or exchange transfusion may be required.

Paracetamol

Hepatic damage, often not evident for several days after ingestion, is a life-threatening complication of overdosage, but fortunately children under age of 10 years are remarkably resistant to the hepatotoxic effects. Vomiting, gastro-intestinal haemorrhage, hyper- or hypoglycaemia, renal tubular damage and cerebral oedema may occur. Management consists of emesis or lavage. Estimate blood paracetamol content 4 hours after ingestion. Patient will require N-acetylcysteine by I.V. infusion if plasma concentration is above a line on a semilogarithmic graph joining 200 μg/ml at 4 hours after ingestion and 30 μg/ml at 15 hours. If in doubt consult Poisons Centre. N-Acetylcysteine (Parvolex) is very effective when given up to 8 hours after overdose. Thereafter its efficacy progressively declines. It is no longer of value by 15 hours and if given at that stage may be harmful.

Iron

The principal effects are gastro-intestinal fluid loss with erosion and haemorrhage, shock and liver damage. The vomit appears rusty (coffee grounds) and has a characteristic metallic smell. Melaena may also be present. The presence of ferrous salts in the vomit can easily be confirmed by the Prussian Blue (ferricyanide) test. The serum iron is raised but does not correlate well with the severity of intoxication.

Treatment is urgent. Give desferrioxamine I.M. then go on to immediate gastric lavage with 1 per cent sodium bicarbonate, some being left in the stomach (see general management).

Desferrioxamine (Desferal) is the specific antidote and should be given in the presence of gastro-intestinal symptoms, shock, altered consciousness or the ingestion of an obviously toxic quantity of iron (e.g. >40 mg elemental iron/kg $\simeq$ 200 mg ferrous sulphate/kg). N.B. *Anaphylaxis* if accidentally given by shot into a vein.

(a) 500 mg to 1 g in 5 ml water is given I.M. as soon as possible (*before lavage*).

(b) 5 g in 50–100 ml water is left in the stomach after lavage.

(c) 15 mg/kg/hour is given I.V. by infusion if the patient is collapsed, the maximum dose being 80 mg/kg/24 hours.

(d) Up to 2 g I.M. may be given 12-hourly if necessary.

Supportive treatment, in particular fluid balance, is vital. In severe cases shock may occur 16–24 hours after ingestion. After recovery severe gastro-intestinal scarring may occur.

Psychotropic Drugs (Barbiturates and other Sedatives)

The chief dangers are respiratory depression and shock.

Hypothermia, water loss from skin and lungs, reduction in urine volume, hypostatic or aspiration pneumonia and cerebral oedema may occur.

Treatment.—The management of pulmonary ventilation and shock comes first. Gastric lavage is usually required but the child who is merely drowsy should be allowed to sleep off the effects under observation. Alkaline osmotic diuresis (see salicylates), dialysis or exchange transfusion may be necessary. Analeptic drugs should not be used.

Tricyclic Antidepressants (Imipramine)

Ingestion of 10 mg/kg or more causes neurological disturbances, respiratory depression and cardiac dysrhythmias. Gastric lavage should be carried out up to 12 hours after ingestion and activated charcoal left in the stomach. Drowsiness occurs, often alternating with periods of excitement, convulsions may be controlled with phenobarbitone or diazepam; if respiratory depression is marked, paraldehyde is preferred. Circulatory collapse may occur up to three days after ingestion. ECG monitoring is essential; atropine-like effects of the drug cause tachycardia, but direct toxic effects on the myocardium may cause ventricular arrhythmias, a-v block, hypotension and QRS changes. Forced diuresis, haemodialysis and haemoperfusion have no place and drug treatment should be avoided if possible in the management of cardiotoxicity. The correction of acidosis by I.V. bicarbonate may restore normal rhythm in children.

Digoxin

Is slowly absorbed and excreted and causes nausea, vomiting, arrhythmias and bradycardia. Management: lavage and then leave activated charcoal in stomach; monitor with ECG and repeated serum potassium for low levels. Bradycardia may require atropine and for arrhythmias give lignocaine/propranolol.

Phenothiazines

Overdosage causes hypotension, hypothermia, tachycardia, cardiac arrhythmias, convulsions, and extrapyramidal reactions. Disturbances of consciousness and respiratory depression are less marked than with other sedatives. The stomach should be emptied using lavage since emetics are of little value in this situation. Treatment is supportive and symptomatic. Severe dyskinesia and oculogyric crisis may be treated with anti-parkinsonian drugs (benztropine mesylate 0·1–0·25 mg I.M.) or antihistamines (e.g. promethazine hydrochloride 1·5 mg/kg I.M.)

Lomotil (diphenoxylate/atropine)

Toxic effects include drowsiness, dizziness, hypo- or hyperthermia and particularly the possibility of cardiorespiratory arrest up to 48 hours after ingestion. Treat by lavage, saline purge and continuous observation for 48 hours. Respiratory depression may require repeated injections of naloxone (Narcan) and possibly artificial ventilation.

Atropine Group

The usual sources are travel sickness pills (hyoscine) and berries (the nightshades). Symptoms are flushed, hot, dry skin, dilated pupils, tachycardia, hyperpyrexia, urinary retention, ataxia, hallucinations, delirium and coma.

Treatment.—Gastric lavage, sedation with chlorpromazine I.M., control of body temperature and high fluid intake. Pilocarpine 0·1 mg/kg I.M. or S.C. will counter the peripheral effects but not the more serious CNS ones.

Amphetamines

Amphetamines cause cerebral stimulation with restlessness, tachycardia, irritability, hallucinations, delirium and convulsions followed by profound depression.

Treatment.—Gastric lavage, activated charcoal and sedation with chlorpromazine. Osmotic diuresis with acidification of the urine to pH 5·3 or less using ammonium chloride 75 mg/kg effectively increases excretion.

Alcohol

Severe hypoglycaemia may develop several hours after the ingestion of alcohol by small children.

Treatment.—Gastric lavage. Oral or intravenous glucose prophylactically. If the blood sugar is low give 30–50 ml 50 per cent dextrose I.V. followed by an I.V. infusion of 20 per cent dextrose.

Household Products (contact Poison Reference Centre)

Caustic alkalis are used in drain cleaners, paint removers and some water softeners. Ingestion causes intensely painful burns of the mouth, pharynx and oesophagus. The mucosa looks soapy white, later becoming brown, oedematous and ulcerated. Perforation of the oesophagus or respiratory obstruction from laryngeal oedema and inability to swallow secretions may occur. Oesophageal stricture may develop after recovery.

Supportive treatment is more important than specific measures. Do NOT perform emesis or lavage (hazard of oesophageal perforation). Attempts to neutralise or dilute the alkali with milk, water, or orange juice are usually unhelpful as the burn is immediate. Oesophagoscopy within 12 hours of injury is advised. If the oesophagus is burnt, broad-spectrum antibiotics should be given and gastrostomy considered. Corticosteroids may prevent the development of a stricture but their use is controversial. Early transfer to a thoracic surgical unit is recommended.

Bleaches are usually solutions of hypochlorites which are corrosives. Give copious milk and 30 ml aluminium hydroxide gel or magnesium hydroxide. The affected skin should be washed thoroughly.

Soaps, detergents and oral contraceptives are mild gastric irritants. Specific treatment is not required.

Disinfectants. Pine-type—emesis, milk and liberal fluids. Phenol type (Lysol and Jeyes' Fluid) rapidly absorbed through skin and mucosae, both of which necrose if untreated. Skin—wash well with alcohol or glycerin. Ingestion: ? lavage (take CARE), then vegetable oil and supportive treatment (beware coma, jaundice, anuria).

Paint

In removing paint from skin and hair, avoid white spirit and other solvents which are themselves harmful to skin and lungs. Instead use animal fat or vegetable oil (e.g. paint-removing cream*) followed by a cetrimide bath. Lead is not a problem in modern household paint but should be considered if industrial paint has been ingested.

---

* For recipe contact the Pharmacy, Birmingham Children's Hospital, Tel. 021 454 4851.

Paraffin (Kerosene, White Spirit) and Petroleum Distillates

Symptoms are due to pulmonary irritation (which can be fatal) and CNS depression.

Do NOT perform emesis or lavage (hazard of aspiration pneumonitis). Liquid paraffin (mineral oil) 50 ml by mouth will delay absorption. Corticosteroids and antibiotics may be of value in lipoid pneumonia.

Paraquat and Diquat

Liquid preparations produce intestinal, renal and hepatic damage and particularly delayed pulmonary fibrosis which is progressive and irreversible. Even small quantities may be lethal and the onset of symptoms delayed for 2–3 days. Urine for analysis (consult Poison Bureau) should be deep-frozen.

Treatment.—SPEED IS ESSENTIAL. Induce vomiting immediately followed by careful gastric lavage. Purge with up to 1 litre 15 per cent Fuller's Earth (adsorbent) including 200 ml 20 per cent mannitol in water which should be given within 30 minutes of ingestion. Continue purgation 2-hourly until stools contain adsorbent. Contact Poisons Reference Centre re further management. Supportive therapy for hepatic and renal failure may be required.

Plants*

Children frequently eat unidentified berries or toadstools. A common example is laburnum seeds which may cause nausea, ataxia, stomach cramps, vomiting, diarrhoea and collapse. Berries of the nightshade family contain hyoscine (see p. 155) and produce dilated pupils, flushing, vomiting, ataxia and hallucinations. Treatment is to empty the stomach and maintain hydration.

Adder Bites

Severe effects are rare and both child and parents should be told this and reassured. They include haemorrhagic and cardiotoxic effects, local pain and swelling, vomiting, colic, diarrhoea, sweating, angioneurotic oedema of lips and tongue, hypotension and renal failure. Management consists of reas-

* See NORTH, P. (1967) *Poisonous Plants and Fungi in Colour*. Poole, Dorset: Blandford Press, and JORDAN, M. (1976) *A Guide to Wild Plants*: the edible and poisonous species of the Northern Hemisphere. London: Millington.

surance, splintage and symptomatic treatment (e.g. paracetamol for pain, chlorpromazine I.M. or I.V. for persistent
vomiting, chlorpheniramine for angioneurotic oedema).

Chart BP, pulse and consciousness level and urine output.
Check ECG, blood urea, cardiac enzymes and WBC count.
Look for systemic bleeding. If no local swelling after 2 hours,
it is unlikely that venom has been transmitted. Observation in
hospital should continue for at least 24 hours.

Antivenom treatment.—Antivenom based on horse serum
is likely to produce anaphylaxis. Its use should only be
considered in the presence of severe life-threatening symptoms, e.g. coma, severe systemic bleeding, persistent or
recurrent hypotension (also ECG changes and WBC
$> 20,000/mm^3$). Zagreb antivenom would be the preferred
product.

Chronic Lead Poisoning

The usual sources are paint, toys and contaminated water,
occasionally the fumes or ashes of burning batteries. Absorbed
lead is deposited mainly in the bones, but the brain, liver and
other viscera may be involved. It is a cumulative poison and
is only slowly removed by treatment.

Symptoms are variable and often insidious. Pallor and pica
are common. Vomiting, anorexia, abdominal pain or constipation may occur. Encephalopathy, common in children, may
present suddenly with convulsions, coma and signs of raised
intracranial pressure or gradually with drowsiness, ataxia,
irritability, overactivity and retarded development.

Investigations.—A raised blood lead of 1·4 μmol/l is
abnormal. Levels above 3 μmol/l should be reduced with
deleading agents. The risk of encephalopathy is great at blood
levels over 4 μmol/l and levels over 5 μmol/l should be treated
urgently. Blood lead estimation is the only diagnostic test but
the following are suggestive: basophil stippling of the red cells
and an iron-deficiency anaemia which is rarely severe. X-rays
show a line of increased density at the metaphyses of the long
bones and X-ray of the abdomen may reveal radio-opaque
material in the gut.

Urinary coproporphyrins and Δ aminolaevulinic acid excretion are increased provided lead has been ingested within
a week of testing. Glycosuria and aminoaciduria (tubular
damage) may occur.

CSF.—Lumbar puncture should be avoided unless necessary for diagnosis. The pressure and protein may be raised. Cells, mainly lymphocytes, are usually below $100/mm^3(100 \times 10^6/1)$.

Treatment.—Should be started as soon as the blood and urine samples have been collected. The removal of residual lead from the gut and the treatment of cerebral oedema are of prime importance, while the establishment of *good urine flow* is essential before chelation is commenced. Proceed as follows:

(1) Treat convulsions and cerebral oedema (see below under Acute encephalopathy).

(2) Remove ingested soluble lead by gastric lavage with dilute magnesium sulphate or sodium sulphate solution or emesis. Do not use purgatives or enemata in the presence of severe symptoms.

(3) Establish good urine flow by infusing 10 per cent dextrose in water I.V. 10–20 ml/kg body weight over a period of 1–2 hours. If urine flow does not start, give mannitol 20 per cent solution 5–10 ml/kg body weight I.V. over 20 minutes. Fluids must be limited to requirements and catheterisation may be necessary in coma. Daily urine output should be 350–500 ml/m²/24 hours. Excessive fluids further increase cerebral oedema.

(4) Chelation. If symptoms of lead poisoning occur, including encephalopathy, start dimercaprol (BAL) 4 mg/kg I.M. 4-hourly for 30 doses. Begin calcium disodium edetate 4 hours later at a separate injection site, 12·5 mg/kg I.M. every 4 hours as 20 per cent solution with 0·5 per cent procaine added, for a total of 30 doses. If there is no obvious improvement by fourth day, increase the number of injections by 10 for each drug. If a good response is obtained and there is no encephalopathy, stop dimercaprol after the third or fourth day and reduce edetate to 50 mg/kg per 24 hours for the remainder of the 5-day course of injections. If blood lead is still above 4 μmol/l 2–3 weeks after the first course, give another 30 injections each of both drugs. Courses of calcium disodium edetate should not exceed 500 mg/kg with at least one week between.

(5) Treat asymptomatic children with blood levels above 5 μmol/l as in (4) if there is intercurrent infection during

convalescence, or if there has been further lead ingestion.

(6) For follow-up care make certain that ingestion of lead does not occur; give penicillamine orally 20 mg/kg daily in 2 doses for 3–6 months or until blood lead falls below 2·9 μmol/l. The maximum dose is 500 mg/day. Give penicillamine on an empty stomach 90 minutes before meal.

General Measures in Acute Encephalopathy

(1) Treat cerebral oedema with mannitol and/or dexamethasone as for status epilepticus (page 124).

(2) Do not use catharsis or enemata in the presence of severe symptoms.

(3) Control convulsions with paraldehyde I.M. (see page 123) or 0·3–0·6 ml/kg rectally diluted with 2 parts vegetable oil. Phenobarbitone, phenytoin and diazepam may increase cerebral oedema and are probably hazardous in the acute stage.

(4) Reduce fever with tepid sponging.

(5) Maintain urine output at 350–500 ml/m²/24 hours with I.V. dextrose avoiding administration of Na-containing fluids.

(6) Withhold oral fluid, food and medication for at least 3 days.

(7) In the presence of impaired renal function, dialysis is mandatory.

M.A.T.

VIII

DIAGNOSIS AND MANAGEMENT OF HAEMATOLOGICAL DISORDERS AND MALIGNANCIES

HAEMORRHAGIC DISORDERS

Screening Tests.—Recommended screening tests for suspected congenital bleeding disorders and prior to visceral biopsy are given on page 165. An appropriate clinical and family history is equally important; in particular, details of the patient's haemostatic response to previous surgical procedures. The ingestion of aspirin and other drugs and vitamin C deficiency should be excluded because a prolonged bleeding time due to abnormal platelet function may result.

Disseminated Intravascular Coagulation.—This may complicate meningococcaemia and septicaemia, newborn hypoxia, extensive surgical procedures, liver failure and other conditions with acidosis and shock. Screening tests which can be performed are given on page 165.

Haemophilia

Diagnosis.—An X-linked recessive disorder occurring in males with a prolonged partial thromboplastin time and normal prothrombin and bleeding times. Factor VIII level is reduced below 50 per cent (0–1 per cent = severe; 1–5 per cent moderately severe; above 5 per cent = mild haemophilia).

Treatment of acute episodes.—Prompt replacement therapy with cryoprecipitate-AHG, freeze-dried factor VIII concentrate within a few hours is vital. Delay overnight may convert a mild bleed into a major one, will retard recovery and also encourage joint damage and muscle wasting. Bed rest, local pressure and haemostatics are of minor importance in comparison. Whenever possible the area should be immobilised (e.g. with a plastic or plaster back slab). Admission is usually required for knee haemarthroses, large haematomas which may cause nerve palsies or vascular obstruction, injuries to the head or mouth and suspected intra-abdominal bleeding. Patients should be screened for hepatitis-associated antigen/antibody.

NEVER cut down, never give aspirin or intramuscular injections, *and never venepuncture the jugular or femoral veins.*

Operative procedures including dental extractions like all other treatment must always be done at Haemophilia Centres because of the need to screen for acquired factor inhibitors and the laboratory monitoring of plasma levels. For dental extractions the F.VIII level should be raised to 50 per cent (confirmed by levels) and the patient started on an antifibrinolytic agent, EACA or tranexamic acid (after eliminating any contra-indications to their use, e.g. haematuria) for 10 days. If bleeding occurs, careful evaluation and further replacement therapy are needed.

For major surgery, the factor level must be raised to 100 per cent and by 12-hourly treatment maintained so that at the trough (i.e. pre next treatment) is 20 per cent or above.

Calculation of dose of factor to be used:

$$\text{No. of units of factor required} = \frac{\text{weight in kg} \times \% \text{ rise required}}{K}$$

where K is the recovery constant.

For F.VIII, $K = 2$ for fresh frozen plasma, 1·5 for cryoprecipitate and 1·5 for F.VIII concentrate.

For F.IX, $K = 0·6$ for concentrate.

Bottles of concentrate will show the number of units they contain and cryoprecipitate contains on average 60–80 units/pack.

The biological half-life of F.VIII is 14 hours and of F.IX 24 hours.

CHRISTMAS DISEASE

Similar to haemophilia in respect of clinical features and inheritance but due to F.IX deficiency. Cryoprecipitate contains no F.IX. Use F.IX concentrate or fresh frozen plasma. For calculation of the dose see above.

VON WILLEBRAND'S DISEASE

An autosomal dominant inherited disorder occurring in homozygous and heterozygous forms, due to defective platelet function because of low VIIIR:AG/VIIIR:WF activity and mild-to-moderate reduction of Factor VIII clotting activity (VIII:C). Haemarthroses are uncommon and mucous membrane bleeding and haematuria are seen more often. Use cryoprecipitate to treat bleeding episodes. Treatment is more complex than for haemophilia and expert advice should be sought.

COAGULATION INVESTIGATIONS

Tests for suspected bleeding disorders

	Normal range
Platelet count	$150–400\times10^9/l$
Bleeding time (Ivy)	up to 7 minutes
Prothrombin time	within 2–3 secs of control
Partial thromboplastin time with kaolin	within 6–7 secs of control
Factor assays	0·50–1·00 units/ml

Screening tests for suspected DIC

	Normal range
Platelet count low*	$150–400\times10^9/l$
Blood film shows red cell fragmentation	
Serial haemoglobin levels*	
P.T. prolonged	within 2–3 secs of control
P.T.T. prolonged	within 6–7 secs of control
Thrombin time prolonged	within 3 secs of control
FDP increased	0–10 μg/ml

* These simple tests are very useful for subsequent assessment of progress.

HAEMOGLOBINOPATHIES

Diagnosis.—Non-Caucasian children (see page 167) should be screened before surgery or if anaemic for the presence of an abnormal haemoglobin by the following tests—haemoglobin level, mean corpuscular volume (MCV), mean corpuscular haemoglobin (MCH), red cell count (RCC) and reticulocyte count, blood film for target cells, solubility test for haemoglobin S, haemoglobin electrophoresis and fetal haemoglobin and haemoglobin A_2 levels (see page 167).

Management

(*a*) **Sickle-cell disease.**—Homozygote (Hb S/S) and double heterozygote (Hb S/C disease, Hb S/Thal) patients should avoid hypoxi , chilling and dehydration. Early treatment of infection ar folic acid supplements are valuable prophylactic measures. When a painful thrombotic crisis develops dehydration should be corrected, any precipitating infection treated, analgesics given, and the patient kept warm. More specific measures (e.g. intravenous magnesium sulphate) are not of proven value when tissue infarction has occurred.

When a surgical procedure under general anaesthesia is required the patient should be pre-oxygenated with 100 per cent oxygen for 5 minutes and the anaesthetic mixture thereafter should contain at least 30 per cent oxygen. Hydration must be maintained with warmed intravenous fluids, hypotension and tourniquets must be avoided, and the patient kept warm. Pre-operative transfusion from the patient's usual haemoglobin level to an arbitrary normal range is not recommended; if transfusion is necessary the blood should be less than 5 days old and warmed during the transfusion. Exchange transfusion should be considered for major procedures.

Sickle-cell heterozygotes (Hb A/S) are unlikely to have symptoms except under conditions of severe hypoxia. Haematuria may occur however.

(*b*) **Hb C, D or E disease.**—The homozygous states of these disorders may cause mild haemolytic anaemia with target cells in the blood film. The heterozygote forms are symptom-free and are not anaemic.

(*c*) **Thalassaemia.**—The β-thalassaemia homozygote (thalassaemia major) is usually dependent on regular transfusions. The haemoglobin level should be maintained above 8·0 g/dl (g/100 ml) using leucocyte-free packed cells. DTPA (2 g) may be added to each unit of blood transfused, but not to exceed a total dose of 6g/transfusion. Daily intramuscular desferrioxamine (500 mg) may be given to delay the onset of transfusion haemosiderosis. Oral iron therapy is contra-indicated but folic acid supplements should be given. Avoid splenectomy unless secondary hypersplenism leads to neutropenia, thrombocytopenia or an increase in transfusion requirements. Check for endocrine effects of excess tissue iron deposition, especially in the pancreas and pituitary.

The β-thalassaemia heterozygote is symptom-free but occasionally shows mild refractory anaemia.

HAEMOGLOBINOPATHIES

Haemoglobin	Geographical origin	Hb level g/dl	Hb electro-phoresis	Fetal Hb level %	Hb A$_2$ level %
Normal (over 1 year)	Any	>10·5	Hb A	<2	<3
Sickle-cell homozygote	African American Caribbean } Negro	5–10	Hb S present Hb A absent	5–10	<3
Sickle-cell heterozygote	Ditto	>10·5	Hb S and Hb A present	<2	<3
Hb S/C disease	Ditto	10–14	Hb S and C present Hb A absent	<2	<3
Sickle/ thalassaemia	Ditto	5–14	Hb S present Hb A absent or much diminished	2–30	<3
Thalassaemia major	Mediterranean countries India Pakistan Middle East Far East Negro	Transfusion dependent	No abnormal haemoglobin	10–90	Up to 7
Thalassaemia minor	Ditto	>10·5 or mild anaemia	No abnormal haemoglobin	Up to 7	Up to 10

G-6-PD DEFICIENCY

This sex-linked disorder may occur in homozygous or heterozygous form in the female or in hemizygous form in the male. It is found in the Mediterranean countries, India, Pakistan, the Middle and Far East and in Negroes. Haemolysis may be induced by drugs and chemicals with oxidant properties and by certain infections. A list of prohibited drugs should be issued to the parents and the general practitioner, and also attached to the hospital case record.

Diagnosis.—There are several screening tests for the detection of glucose-6-phosphate dehydrogenase (G-6-PD) deficiency; a positive result should then be confirmed by a spectrophotometric assay of the actual G-6-PD level.

Drugs and Other Agents available in the U.K. which may cause Haemolysis in Children with Red Cell Glucose-6-Phosphate Dehydrogenase (G-6-PD) Deficiency:

Analgesics and Antipyretics
    acetylsalicylic acid (aspirin)   phenacetin (acetophenetidin)
    *phenazone (antipyrine)

Antimalarials
    chloroquine   mepacrine   primaquine

Antibiotics
    chloramphenicol   nalidixic acid   niridazole   PAS
    nitrofurans   sulphonamides   sulphones

Diabetic Acidosis

Infections
    Miscellaneous bacterial and viral infections (e.g. pneumonia, hepatitis, mononucleosis).
    When infections in G-6-PD deficient patients have been treated with chemotherapeutic agents it may be difficult to establish whether the infection or the chemotherapeutic agent precipitated haemolysis.

Miscellaneous agents
    dichloralphenazone   dimercaprol   *fava beans
    methylene blue   naphthalene   probenecid   *quinidine
    vitamin C (ascorbic acid)   vitamin K_1 (large doses of water-soluble preparations)

  * Reported to cause haemolysis in G-6-PD deficient Caucasians but not in deficient Negroes.

ROUTINE HAEMATOLOGICAL VALUES
approximate normal range

Age	Hb g/dl (g/100 ml)	PCV	WCC ×10⁹/l	Neutrophils %	MCV fl	MCHC %
Cord blood	13·5–20·0	0·50–0·56	9–30	50–80	110–128	29·5–33·5
day 1	17·0–21·0	0·55–0·65	9–40	50–80	110–128	29·5–33·5
day 4	16·0–20·0	0·50–0·58	6–20	35–60	107–121	31 –34
week 2	14·5–18·0	0·50–0·55	6–15	30–50	100–120	30 –34
6 months	10·0–12·5	0·33–0·38	6–15	30–50		
1–5 years	10·5–13·0	0·36–0·40	6–15	30–50	80–96	32 –36
5–10 years	11·0–14·0	0·37–0·42	5–15	40–65		
10–15 years	11·5–14·5	0·38–0·42	4–13	50–75		

Serum B$_{12}$ 150–1000 ng/l ⎫ 5 ml in plain tube
Serum folate   3·0–20 ng/ml ⎭
Red cell folate   100–640 ng/ml   2 ml in heparin or sequestrene tube.

Transfusion of Blood Products.
The infant's blood volume is 8 per cent (80 ml/kg) of the body weight, so that a whole blood transfusion of 20 ml/kg will raise the haemoglobin by approximately 25 per cent.
Amount of packed cells required (ml) = Wt (kg)×3×desired rise in Hb (g/dl).
The maximum rates recommended for the treatment of coagulation disorders or for transfusing anaemic patients (e.g. thalassaemics and leukaemics) but not for those being transfused after acute haemorrhage, are:
(a) Fresh frozen plasma 20 ml per kg in 30 minutes
(b) Whole blood ⎫ 2·5 ml per kg per hour
(c) Packed cells ⎭ Maximum in one transfusion 50 ml per kg
Platelet concentrate: 1 unit = platelet concentrate from one pint of blood.
1 unit/m² raises platelet count by 10×10⁹/l.
To arrest haemorrhage due to thrombocytopenia give at least 4 units/m².

F.G.H.H.

MALIGNANCIES

Diagnosis

Extensive diagnostic resources are required for managing children with cancer as approximately one-third have leukaemia, one-third have CNS tumours and the remainder have a variety of rare solid tumours. Therefore whenever possible children with suspected cancer should be referred to a specialist paediatric oncology centre for investigation and treatment.

Leukaemia should always be confirmed by bone marrow aspirate and the cell type determined by cytochemical, immunological and other techniques; approximately 80 per cent are lymphoblastic and about 20 per cent acute myeloid; both groups include sub-types with important therapeutic implications.

For solid tumours facilities must be available for arteriography, ultrasonography, CT scanning, lymphangiography, for detecting specific tumour markers such as urinary catecholamines which are elevated in neuroblastoma patients and serum alphafetoprotein (elevated in hepatoma and some teratoma patients). The paediatric histopathologist should be consulted before the biopsy since special techniques may be needed, e.g. immunological studies for lymphoma tissue diagnosis, or electron microscopy.

Treatment—General Points

Most paediatric tumours respond to cytotoxic drugs which, with appropriate surgery and radiotherapy, have greatly improved the chances of cure. The optimal combinations of treatments are still under investigation by clinical trials organised by the Medical Research Council, the United Kingdom Children's Cancer Study Group and other bodies. Accurate classification and staging are essential.

At diagnosis and following chemo- or radiotherapy the patient may have severe metabolic or nutritional problems and is at risk of septicaemia and/or bleeding. Take blood cultures when febrile, especially if neutropenic, and use a broad-spectrum antibiotic combination immediately if there is any suspicion of infection. Intramuscular injections must not be given in the presence of thrombocytopenia. When there is severe thrombocytopenia and bleeding give platelet concentrates (see p. 169). Occasionally white cell concentrates are needed for severe infections in neutropenic patients not responding to antibiotics. Pay careful attention to fluid balance and nutrition; special diets or parental nutrition may be needed.

Allopurinol to prevent uric acid nephropathy may be needed in the first few days of cytotoxic treatment when rapid breakdown of malignant cells occurs. Do not give allopurinol with 6-mercaptopurine as it prevents metabolism of the 6MP.

Plot blood counts and treatments on semi-logarithmic haematology charts available from Wightman Mountain Ltd, 32–34 Great Peter Street, London, SW1. Reference No. BMJ 22870. Stop treatment if platelet count is <100 or neutrophil count $<1 \cdot 0 \times 10^9/1$.

Varicella and measles may be fatal. If contact with these occurs, give within 72 hours for varicella, zoster immune globulin 1 g/m² I.M. and for measles, pooled human gamma-globulin 1 g/m² I.M.

Grave emotional and psychological stresses affect children with cancer and their families, and social worker support is usually needed.

Terminal care requires skilled attention. For analgesia, oral morphine 3–4-hourly is effective if given regularly in adequate dose; the drug may be given subcutaneously if the child cannot swallow.

CYTOTOXIC DRUGS

These are very dangerous as they can all cause bone marrow aplasia and many have other adverse effects. All doses should be checked against the patient's treatment protocol and be calculated using the child's surface area. When in doubt consult the senior registrar or consultant on call. Take the following precautions when giving intravenous drugs:

- (a) Avoid contamination of your skin and eyes—wear plastic or rubber gloves, and glasses if possible.
- (b) Have hydrocortisone and equipment for resuscitation available.
- (c) Check all doses and diluents with another doctor or a trained nurse before administration.

(d) Give I.V. drugs via butterfly needle. Flush approximately 3 ml normal saline through first to confirm the needle is in the vein, then change to syringe containing drug. Afterwards flush vein with more saline.

(e) Do not mix drugs.

(f) Give adequate anti-emetics before administering drugs which may cause vomiting.

Actinomycin D	Strongly corrosive if extravasated. Emetic. Overdoses are usually fatal.
Adriamycin (Doxorubicin)	Ditto. Also cardiotoxic so give slowly over 3–5 minutes, well diluted. Do not exceed 450 mg/m² cumulative dose.
Asparaginase	Anaphylaxis may occur. Observe patient for at least 30 minutes after dose. May cause pancreatitis and liver damage.
Bleomycin	Risk of pulmonary fibrosis. Do not exceed 360 mg/m² cumulative dose.
Cis-platinum	Emetic and nephrotoxic. Check renal function before each dose, pre-hydrate and after dose give forced diuresis (see detailed instructions).
Cyclophosphamide	Emetic. I.V. hydration for several hours required after large I.V. doses to prevent haemorrhagic cystitis.
Cytosine arabinoside	Emetic. If given intrathecally, dilute with normal saline 100 mg to 10 ml, *not* diluent supplied with drug.
Daunorubicin (Rubidomycin)	Emetic, corrosive and cardiotoxic. Give slowly over 3–5 minutes well diluted. Do not exceed 300 mg/m² cumulative dose.
DTIC (imidazole carboxamide)	Decomposes on exposure to light. Wrap syringe in foil to exclude light and use immediately.
Methotrexate	May cause gastro-intestinal ulceration. Specific antidote is folinic acid which should be given I.V. 24 mg/m² 8-hourly to reverse severe toxicity. For high-dose regimens with folinic acid rescue, good renal function and hydration are essential—see detailed protocol. For intrathecal use administer special preservative-free preparation.
Mustine	Emetic and corrosive. Give in fast-running drip.
Vinblastine	Corrosive
Vincristine	Corrosive and neurotoxic. Give aperient to prevent constipation and colic.

Prognosis

This has greatly improved for many tumours, although some children have residual handicaps and a few will develop second malignancies, infertility and other late-effects. In assessing the likelihood of cure the clinical stage and other prognostic features at presentation in the individual patient must be taken into account as well as 5-year survival rates for children with the tumour concerned, e.g. 25–50 per cent for acute lymphoblastic leukaemia, 80–90 per cent for Hodgkin's disease, 65–95 per cent for nephroblastoma, 25–50 per cent for CNS tumours, 40–60 per cent for osteogenic sarcoma, 60–90 per cent for rhabdomyosarcomas.

J.R.M.

[NOTES]

IX
CLINICAL CHEMISTRY

REFERENCE INTERVALS FOR ENZYME ACTIVITIES

Enzyme	E.C. No.*	Range (U/l)		Comments
Alanine aminotransferase	2.6.1.2.	less than 40[+]		
Alkaline phosphatase	3.1.3.1.	Newborns	150–600[+]	highest at birth
		6–24m	250–1000	
		2–5y	250–850	
		6–7y	250–1000	
		8–9y	250–750	
		10–11y females 250–950 males 250–730		
		12–13y females 200–730 males 275–785		
		14–15y females 170–460 males 170–970		
		16–18y females 75–270 males 125–720		
		18y females 60–250 males 50–200		
Aspartate aminotransferase	2.6.1.1.	less than 40[+]		
Amylase	3.2.1.1.	70–300**		pre-pubertal females
Creatine kinase	2.7.3.2.	males—less than 80[++]		same as males
				higher at birth
γ-Glutamyl transferase	2.3.2.2.	less than 20		

NOTE: Large variations in ranges can occur depending upon methodology.

* E.C. No. = enzyme commission number

** Pharmacia Diagnostics A.B.

[+] Scandinavian Society for Clinical Chemistry and Clinical Physiology recommendation 1975

[++] Midland Centre for Neurosurgery and Neurology (see also p. 210).

AVERAGE BIOCHEMICAL REFERENCE INTERVALS FOR HEALTHY CHILDREN

Specimen. The material preferred for analysis is indicated in brackets: B = whole blood; P = plasma; S = serum.
* Denotes those investigations often collected by laboratory staff or where special preparation or precautions are needed before collecting the specimen.
Concentrations of sodium and potassium in some specimens of capillary blood may be increased to a variable extent.

Blood	S.I. Units		Conventional Units (and Conversion factor)		Comments
Acid base (Astrup, B)*					Values for arterial blood;
pH (Hydrogen ion)	7·36–7·42 (38–44 nmol/l)		—		results from capillary blood from *warmed* limb are similar.
Pco₂	4·3–6·1	kPa	32–46	mmHg (0·133)	
Standard bicarbonate	21–25	mmol/l	—		
Base excess	−2–+2	mmol/l	—		Newborn period, down to −4 mmol/l.
Po₂ (arterial)	11·3–14·0	kPa	85–105	mmHg (0·133)	
α-1-antitrypsin	1·4–3·4	g/l	—		—if deficient P₁-typing of family recommended[1]
Ammonium nitrogen (Fenton method, P)*	2–25	μmol/l	3–35	μg/dl (0·714)	Newborn period, twice as high.
Bilirubin, Total (P, S.)	2–16	μmol/l	0·1–0·8	mg/dl (17·1)	
Calcium (P, S)	2·25–2·75	mmol/l	9–11	mg/dl (0·25)	Newborn period, lower. Avoid venous stasis.
Cholesterol (P.S) (fasting)	2·6–5·7	mmol/l	100–200	mg/dl (0·0259)	Lower in first year.
Creatinine (P. S)	25–115	μmol/l	0·3–1·3	mg/dl (88·4)	Increases with age within this range.
Electrolytes (P, S)					
Sodium	136–145	mmol/l	—		
Potassium	4·0–5·5	mmol/l	—		
Chloride	98–105	mmol/l	—		
Glucose (specific, fasting) (P, B)	2·5–5·3	mmol/l	45–95	mg/dl (0·0555)	Lower in newborn period.

	S.I. Units	Conventional Units (and Conversion factor)		Comments
Blood				
Iron (S)	9–36	μmol/l	50–200	μg/dl	(0·179)	High in newborn period, increases with age.
Iron-binding capacity (S)	estimate transferrin			
Lead (B)	less than 1·75	μmol/l	less than 36	μg/dl	(0·0484)	
Magnesium (P, S)	0·6–1·0	mmol/l	1·5–2·5	mg/dl	(0·411)	
Osmolality (P, S)	275–295	mosmol/kg	—		
Phenylalanine (P)	0·04–0·21	mmol/l	0·7–3·5	mg/dl	(0·0605)	Higher in newborn period. Upper limit 25% lower in older children.
Phosphate, inorganic (as P) (P, S)	1·1–1·9	mmol/l	3·5–6·0	mg/dl	(0·323)	
Protein (S)				
Total	63–81	g/l		
Albumin	36–48	g/l	—	
Globulin	23–37	g/l	—	
Immunoglobulins				
IgA	0·8–4·5	g/l	—		IgA—Low at birth, rises gradually to adult levels during childhood.
IgG	5–18	g/l	adult levels		IgG—High at birth, decreases during first 4m, rises to adult levels during first 5y.
IgM	0·2–2·0	g/l	—		IgM—Low at birth, rises to adult levels during first year.
IgE	less than 100–500 I.U./ml			
Transferrin	2·5–4·5	g/l		
Triglyceride (S)* (fasting)	0·34–1·92	mmol/l	30–170	mg/dl	(0·0113)	
Urate (P, S)	0·12–0·36	mmol/l	2–6	mg/dl	(0·0595)	
Urea (fasting) (P, S)	2·5–6·6	mmol/l	15–40	mg/dl	(0·166)	
Faeces				
Fat (as stearic acid)	less than 16·2 mmol/day		less than 4·5 g/day	(3·52)	
Cerebrospinal fluid				
Protein (Total)	0·2–0·4	g/l		
Glucose	2·5–4·8	mmol/l	45–85	mg/dl	—	CSF glucose should equal or exceed ¾ × blood glucose.

CLINICAL CHEMISTRY

General

Blood specimens, clotted (to yield serum), fluoride-oxalate (for glucose) and heparinised (whole blood or plasma) are usually suitable. For bilirubin, the specimen must be kept in the dark. Many analyses (electrolytes and enzymes) require prompt separation of cells from plasma.

Urine specimens may require appropriate preservatives. 24-hour collections should be complete and even trivial losses reported. The duration of shorter collections should be governed by the times the patient passes urine (noted exactly) rather than by the clock.

Acid-Base Balance (Astrup)

Venous samples are unsuitable. Provided there is good peripheral flow, achieved by warming the limb if necessary, capillary blood is suitable. Blood from an arterial catheter may be taken in a heparinised syringe without entrapment of air and the syringe closed by a cap or bending the needle back. The specimen must then be delivered without delay to the laboratory. When abnormal, the patient's rectal temperature should be reported to enable an approximate correction of the results to be made. Results are reported as pH (or hydrogen ion concentration [H^+]), Pco_2, standard bicarbonate and base excess. The Pco_2 measures the respiratory component of acid-base balance. Standard bicarbonate, which is the concentration of bicarbonate in fully oxygenated whole blood when the Pco_2 is 5·3 kPa (40 mmHg) and the temperature 37°C, measures the non-respiratory component. Base excess (which may be negative) is derived from the standard bicarbonate. This may be used to assess the base required for whole body correction, which is equal to the base excess in mmol/l×body weight in kg×0·3. (The total required is greater than this but the amount derived from this formula will avoid transient dangerously high blood levels.)

RELATIONSHIP OF pH TO HYDROGEN ION (H⁺) CONCENTRATION

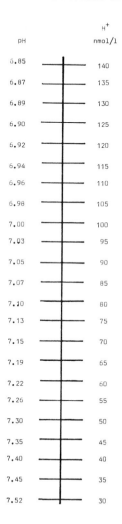

pH | H^+ nmol/l

Approximate reference values
38–44 nmol/l.

Notes
1. Ideally, arterial blood taken anaerobically in a heparinised syringe is required. *Free flowing* capillary blood, collected carefully in special tubes, may also be used.
2. Blood *must* be taken to the laboratory promptly.
3. For text see page 180.

GASTRO-INTESTINAL FUNCTION

COMMONER CAUSES OF DIARRHOEA AND MALABSORPTION

1. **Persistent post-infective diarrhoea** in young infants is frequently associated with secondary lactase deficiency leading to lactose intolerance. Stools contain fluid which is acid and positive for reducing substances (see below). Severe cases may also be intolerant of monosaccharides as well.

Specific inborn errors of sugar absorption as a cause of fluid diarrhoea are rare, i.e. specific lactase deficiency, sucrase-isomaltase deficiency, glucose-galactose malabsorption.

Note that carbohydrate malabsorption may cause diarrhoea by bacterial degradation of unabsorbed sugar to short-chain fatty acids, in which case there may be no detectable carbohydrate in the stool.

2. **Cow's milk protein intolerance** which may be associated with secondary lactose intolerance. Withdrawal of milk protein with return of symptoms on milk challenge is the only reliable diagnostic test. The challenge should be conducted under close supervision with small volumes of milk (initially 1 ml or less) if the infant is thought to be very sensitive to cow's milk.

3. **Coeliac disease** or permanent gluten intolerance. Minimum diagnostic criteria are an abnormal upper small bowel mucosal histology demonstrated by peroral biopsy and good clinical response to gluten-free diet (see page 41). Peroral biopsy is a safe procedure in experienced hands even in small infants, with the exception of those who are very marasmic. However, it should be restricted to centres where sufficient experience is constantly gained to ensure both the minimum of technical difficulties for the patient's benefit, and correct interpretation of findings.

4. **Cystic fibrosis.**—Suspected from association of chronic respiratory symptoms with failure to thrive and bulky stools with an offensive *penetrating* odour.

The sweat test is the most definitive test (see below).

Approximately 90 per cent of C.F. patients have pancreatic insufficiency and therefore steatorrhoea. Examination of stools for fat globules is usually sufficient to demonstrate this and fat balance or duodenal intubation is only necessary in doubtful cases.

DETAILS OF TESTS

Stool microscopy—Cysts and ova indicate infestation with protozoa (giardia lamblia) or worms. Giardial infestation may be present even in absence of cysts in stool—motile forms can be seen in warm duodenal fluid or from jejunal biopsy smears.

Stool pH.—Test *fluid* part of stool with pH indicator paper—pH 5·5 or less is abnormal and usually indicates sugar malabsorption (colonic bacteria ferment sugars to lactic acid).

Reducing substances in stool.—Use freshly passed stool and examine fluid part (collection will require plastic napkin liner or other manoeuvre). Mix 2 vol. water to 1 vol. faeces. Place 15 drops of mixture in tube and add 1 Clinitest tablet. Read colour on Clinitest chart. Quarter per cent or less is negative; $\frac{1}{4}$–$\frac{1}{2}$ per cent suspect; $\frac{1}{2}$ per cent or more is positive for reducing sugar (e.g. lactose or monosaccharides, glucose, galactose or fructose) and suggests sugar intolerance. For demonstration of sucrose dilute HCl should be added to stool mixture which is then boiled before Clinitest tablet is added.

Faecal fat excretion (quantitative).—Collect all stools for three consecutive days. If stools are passed irregularly and days are missed, the collection should be extended for a fourth or fifth day. In children over 6 months of age a normal average daily excretion on an adequate intake of fat for age should not exceed 14 mmol (4 g) per day. It is necessary to estimate the intake of fat accurately.

Raised fat excretion is a reliable index of malabsorption but does not differentiate underlying pathology.

One-hour blood xylose method (infants and children under 30 kg).—Following a fast of at least 6 hours, the patient is given 5 g of D-xylose, in 100 ml of water. Exactly one hour later, 1–2 ml of venous blood is taken into a standard fluoride (blood sugar) tube. A one-hour blood level above 1·3 mmol/l (20 mg/100 ml) is normal. A result below this is abnormal but should be confirmed by a repeat test the next day.

The one-hour blood xylose level indicates rate of absorption in the upper gut and is abnormal when the mucosal brush border is damaged.

Sweat test using pilocarpine iontophoresis. Na and Cl levels above 60 mmol/l denote cystic fibrosis provided at least 100 mg of sweat is obtained and the difference between Na and Cl is less than 30 mmol/l. If the individual values lie between 45 and 75 the test should be repeated. It is reliable from the age of six weeks; small infants should be well wrapped and two gauze swabs used simultaneously.

RENAL FUNCTION

Renal function may be measured in terms of (1) excretory capacity, which is reflected by the glomerular filtration rate (GFR); (2) tubular function, which is subdivided into (i) proximal tubular reabsorption, (ii) regulation of acid-base balance and (iii) handling of water; and (3) the presence of abnormalities such as protein and cells. In most forms of acute and chronic renal disease, defects in tubular function will roughly parallel the impairment of GFR, and it is not ordinarily necessary to assess them separately. Detailed studies may be required in the assessment of metabolic acidosis, polyuria/polydypsia and familial rickets, but the techniques are outside the scope of this volume, with the exception of the urine concentration test, which may conveniently be combined with the measurement of proteinuria.

Endogenous creatinine clearance.—The height and weight of the patient must be notified to the laboratory. The collections of urine must be complete in volume and accurate in timing. Their duration should be determined by the voiding of urine and not by the clock.

Normal activity, diet and fluid intake are encouraged on the day before the test. On the day of the test the child should remain reclining. Breakfast should be light, avoiding meat protein. If it is necessary for the continued co-operation of the patient, milk or a biscuit may be given.

To ensure the adequate flow of urine (approx. 2 ml/min/m²) a minimum of 10 ml/kg water, flavoured if desired, should be given during the hour before the test. During the test, fluid should be given at half this rate (i.e. 5 ml/kg) or more if the diuresis is inadequate, drinks being given at approximately half-hourly intervals.

At about 09.00 h patient empties bladder completely, and the urine is discarded and the time recorded. All urine that is now passed up to approximately 12.00 h is collected and combined as specimen A. The nearest time to 12.00 h of voiding the last specimen is recorded and this ends the first collection.

At about 12.00 h blood is taken for analysis and sent straight to the laboratory. All urine passed after the end of the first collection and up to and including a specimen passed at about 15.00 h is collected and combined as specimen B. The time of voiding this last specimen is recorded accurately. This allows two separate calculations of clearance to be made. If these do not agree the test is repeated.

The mean normal value for endogenous creatinine clearances is 123 ($\pm$20 per cent) ml/min/1·73 m² body surface area. In very young children, lower values may be normal, e.g. 36 ml/min/1·73 m² at one week. This test suffers from a number of inherent disadvantages: (i) with normal or mildly impaired GFR, small differences in the already low plasma creatinine concentration are not easily determined; (ii) stasis in the lower urinary tract, from reflux, obstruction or neurogenic bladder, may cause major bladder-emptying errors; and (iii) the accuracy of timed urine collections may be influenced by human error. Catheterisation is an unacceptable solution.

Clearance of ⁵¹Chromium-labelled edetic acid (⁵¹Cr EDTA).—If facilities for the dispensing and measurement of radio-isotopes are available this test gives a more reliable measure of GFR than endogenous creatinine clearance. This substance is handled exclusively by the glomerulus and the principle of the technique is to inject a measured dose intravenously, allow time for equilibration between the plasma and extracellular fluid, and then calculate the rate of disappearance of radioactivity from the plasma by means of two or three blood samples, appropriately spaced. Elimination of the need for timed urine collections has distinct advantages.

The pharmacy prepares the dose of ⁵¹Cr EDTA to be administered containing 1·0 μCi per kg body weight (if GFR is estimated to be greater than 80 ml/min/1·73 m² then only half the dose is prepared). Draw all but 0·15 ml into a syringe, leaving the 0·15 ml in the bottle to be sent to the laboratory for use as the standard. Inject the ⁵¹Cr EDTA intravenously as quickly as possible and wash through with 5 ml of 0·9 per cent saline, recording the time. Blood samples (5 ml in lithium heparin) should preferably be taken from a different vein to avoid radioactive contamination. The standard, the syringes and the blood specimens are all sent to the laboratory for analysis. The latter are taken at the following intervals: 2, 4 and 6 hours if the estimated GFR is less than 30; 2 and 4 hours if GFR is estimated to be between 30–60; and 2 and 3 hours if greater than 60 ml/min/1·73 m². A crude estimate of the GFR can be determined from the following formula:

$$GFR = \frac{49\cdot5 \times \text{height (cm)}}{\text{plasma creatinine } (\mu\text{mol/l})}$$

The constant used will vary according to the method of determination of creatinine; the one quoted is for the kinetic Jaffé method.

Overnight urine collection.—This test is carried out during enforced fluid restriction and affords a screening test for renal concentrating ability as well as a means of measuring protein-uria. Since the urine is secreted during recumbency, the test can be used to distinguish postural from fixed proteinuria, while it also causes less inconvenience than a 24 h collection.

The child is not allowed to drink after 16.00–17.00 h on the evening of the test. A dry supper with ample protein content should be taken. At bedtime the bladder is emptied and the urine discarded. The exact time is recorded. On waking the bladder is again emptied and all the urine is collected, the time again being recorded. Any urine passed during the night must also be saved. The whole collection is sent to the laboratory, together with the patient's weight and height, from which surface area may be calculated. The urine volume and its protein content are measured, and the protein excretion rate is expressed as mg/h/m². The upper limit of normal is 4 mg/h/m²; heavy proteinuria is usually defined as > 40 mg/h/m².

If the fluid intake has been adequately restricted, the osmolality of the collection should reach 800 mosmol/kg. Failure to do so, in the absence of impaired GFR, would indicate the need for a full water deprivation test.

Water deprivation test.—Weigh the patient and be prepared to assess clinical dehydration by further weighing, and if necessary discontinue the test. Collect urine and blood for baseline osmolality determination. At 18.00 h give the patient a dry supper with ample protein content and a small amount of fluid not exceeding 150 ml. Prohibit all food and further fluid until the test has been completed. Collect all further urine samples separately through the night and following morning until the osmolality is constant and check that at least 3 per cent loss in weight has occurred. The test should be stopped if weight loss reaches 5 per cent.

In unimpaired renal function, at least one urine specimen will have an osmolality over 800 mosmol/kg and the plasma osmolality will remain normal (275–295 mosmol/kg). In severe renal failure the osmolality is less than 300 mosmol/kg and the plasma osmolality may be greater than normal. In diabetes insipidus the osmolality rarely exceeds 100 mosmol/kg. With moderate impairment of renal function the highest urine osmolality will lie between these values.

K.D.G.
R.H.R.W.

TESTS OF ENDOCRINE FUNCTION

NOMENCLATURE AND ABBREVIATIONS

Introduction of SI units and new tests of endocrine function have led to confusion in some areas of Paediatric Endocrinology. This is particularly so in the use of abbreviations. Some abbreviations are universally accepted, others are not. The following list of abbreviations and, where appropriate, their synonyms, are offered as a guide. If in doubt, please consult your local Endocrine Laboratory.

Abbreviations in brackets are acceptable when requesting assays.

Trophic Hormones

Trophic-stimulating hormones are produced at pituitary level. These are:
- (*a*) Adrenocorticotrophin, corticotrophin (ACTH).
- (*b*) Thyrotrophin (TSH).
- (*c*) Follicle-stimulating hormone (FSH).
- (*d*) Luteinizing hormone (LH). Sometimes, ICSH, interstitial cell-stimulating hormone.
- (*e*) Growth hormone (hGH).
- (*f*) Prolactin—no abbreviation acceptable.

Releasing Hormones (Releasing Factors)

Releasing hormones (RH) arise at hypothalamic level and increase the production of trophic hormones. At least two are fully characterised and synthesised. The abbreviation (RH) is preferred to RF (releasing factor) in view of the well-documented "hormonal" effects, except where characterisation is incomplete.
- (*a*) Corticotrophin-releasing hormone (factor) (CRF).
- (*b*) Luteinising and follicle-stimulating hormone-releasing hormone (LH-RH or LH-FSH-RH), sometimes less correctly referred to as LRF.
- (*c*) Thyrotrophin-releasing hormone (TRH), sometimes less correctly TRF.

Hormones and their Reference Values

Serum is required for all hormone analyses in blood. 2 ml serum (minimum of 1·0 ml) for *each* estimation requested should be collected. The basal values quoted are those obtained from hospitalised and non-hospitalised children and adults in whom no endocrine abnormality was demonstrable. The concentrations cited are those calculated for 95 per cent confidence limits in most cases. When the data is not normally distributed a mean or range is quoted.

NORMAL VALUES

It is important to note that for peptide hormones the nationally or internationally approved standards are used to calculate the values. The current standard employed for each peptide hormone is quoted in parentheses after the reference value. These standards may change from time to time according to international agreements on biological standards. Consult your local laboratory if in doubt.

Steroid hormone concentrations, especially testosterone and oestradiol, are related to sexual maturation and the sex of the patient. Values quoted should be carefully assessed in relation to the clinical picture, sex and maturation in all cases.

The following published references will be useful when seeking values for hormones reported by other laboratories using similar techniques employed locally.

(1) *Paediatric Chemical Pathology*. B. E. Clayton, P. Jenkins & J. M. Round. Published by Blackwells, Oxford, 1980.
(2) *Specialised assay services for hospital laboratories, provided by the Supraregional Assay Service (SAS)*, 3rd edition, Professor S. R. Stitch (Ed.), printed by University of Leeds (1980). See local laboratory for details.

Peptide Hormones in Serum
TSH
1–5 mU/l (MRC 68/38) pre- and full-term infants show a rapid increase in TSH during the first few hours and days (20–50 mU/l), returning to normal at 5 days.

hGH (Mean values)
< 5 mU/l (MRC 66/217)
After insulin induced hypoglycaemia (IIH) one value at least > 15 mU/l.
After prolonged glucose tolerance test (PGTT) one value at least > 20 mU/l.

Prolactin
    Children up to puberty (both sexes)
    114–383 mU/l (MRC 75/704)
    Note: prolactin is a "stress" hormone and may rise above
    the values quoted in a severely distressed child.

LH
Children 6m	1–18 I.U./l (MRC 68/40)
Children 6m–10y	< 1–8 I.U./l (MRC 68/40)
Adult males	1–8 I.U./l (MRC 68/40)
Adult females	
(luteal/follicular)	1–12 I.U./l (MRC 68/40)

FSH
Children 6m	1–4 U/l (MRC 78/549)
Children 6m–10y	< 1–3 U/l (MRC 78/549)
Adult males	1–7 U/l (MRC 78/549)
Adult females	
luteal/follicular)	1–9 U/l (MRC 78/549)

Note: Children in whom pubertal development is well
    advanced, may show increased FSH values, similar to
    adults. Girls at menarche may show typical cyclic varia-
    tions as for adult females.

Steroid Hormones in Serum
Gonadal steroids

Testosterone
Prepubertal girls and boys	0·1–1·0 nmol/l
Adult females	0·8–3·0 nmol/l
Adult males	11·00–36·0 nmol/l

Note: Values for testosterone in boys rise steadily through-
    out puberty reaching the lower adult male limits by
    Tanner pubertal stage IV.

Oestradiol-17 β
    Data is sparse for prepubertal children, but best estimates
    suggest values are similar to adult males.
Adult males	120–180 pmol/l
Adult females (follicular)	160–1310 pmol/l
Adult females (luteal)	220–1480 pmol/l

Adrenal cortex
  Cortisol (both sexes)
   (a.m.)   200–700 nmol/l (range)
  *(p.m.) < 140 nmol/l (mean)
  * Based on values from unstressed patients at midnight.
  Lack of diurnal rhythm may be indicative of Cushing's
  disease (see below under Circadian Rhythm in tests of
  adrenal function).

Dehydroepiandrosterone sulphate (DHAS)
  Useful index of hyperplasia or suspected androgen-
  secreting tumour.
  Infants (5–11 days)   0·8–2·8 μmol/l (range)
  Children (5–15 years)   0·1–3·6 μmol/l (range)
  Adult males (18–49 years)   5–9·9 μmol/l (range)
  Adult females (21–35 years)   2·7–8·7 μmol/l (range)

  Note: DHAS is the principal androgen secreted by the
    adrenal cortex.

17α-hydroxyprogesterone (17-OHP)
  Indications: In diagnosis of Congenital Adrenal Hyper-
    plasia (CAH) 21 hydroxylase deficiency.
  Neonates (5–11 days, full term)   1·6–7·5 nmol/l (range)
  Children (4–15 years)   0·4–4·2 nmol/l (range)
  Adult females (follicular)   1·0–2·7 nmol/l (range)
  Adult females (luteal)   4·5–16·1 nmol/l (range)
  Adult males   1·7–3·8 nmol/l (range)

  Note: There is a rapid fall from very high levels of 17-
    OHP maternal source in first 24–48 h of life. This is an
    inappropriate time to measure 17-OHP for diagnostic
    purposes. Premature infants also have 2–3 fold higher
    levels of 17-OHP compared with values quoted for full-
    term infants.

Urinary steroids
  11-oxygenation index. (Ratio of pregnanetriol to cortisol
    metabolism.) A useful index for diagnosing congenital
    adrenal hyperplasia. If monitoring of adequacy of sub-
    stitution therapy is required, request pregnanetriol excre-

tion on a 24 h urine. A value of 3 μmol/day favours adequacy of therapy.

Random urine sample (40 ml) collection without preservative. Normal value < 0·5.

Note: Urine should always accompany requests for serum 17-OHP.

Free cortisol in urine

< 30–350 nmol/24 h

Note: There is a positive correlation of basal urinary cortisol with body weight in children. To an approximation, basal values are 2·8–8·4 nmol/kg.

TESTS OF ADRENAL FUNCTION

Synacthen test (short)

Indications: Screening test for adrenal insufficiency.

Assay request: serum cortisol.

Patient preparation: none.

Drug: Tetracosactrin (Synacthen) 250 micrograms at 0 time.

Procedure: Collect basal (0) sample (09.00–10.00 h), inject Synacthen and collect further samples at 30 and 60 minutes.

Synacthen test (long)

Indications: Test for primary adrenal insufficiency.

Assay request: serum cortisol.

Patient preparation: none.

Drug: Tetracosactrin (Synacthen Depot) 0·5 mg I.M. twice-daily for 4 days commencing 0 time.

Procedure: Collect basal (0) sample (09.00–10.00 h), give first injection (09.00–10.00 h) and repeat at 18.00 h. Repeat injection schedule each day and collect samples at 24, 48, 72 and 96 h.

Circadian Rhythm (cortisol)

Indications: Investigation of Cushing's syndrome. Normal response: at least a 50 per cent fall at 24.00 h compared to 09.00 h.

Assay request: serum cortisol.

Patient preparation: hospitalised, indwelling venous catheter (older patients). Patient asleep for 24.00 h specimen.
Drug: none.
Procedure: Collect serum sample on day 1 at 24.00 h; day 2 at 09.00 h.

Dexamethasone screening test
Indications: Investigation of Cushing's syndrome.
Note: A circadian rhythm (see above) should precede this investigation to obtain basal values.
Assay request: serum cortisol.
Patient preparation: none.
Drug: Dexamethasone tablets 1 mg (or 2 mg if 20 per cent over ideal body weight) at 22.00 h on day 1.
Procedure: Collect serum sample at 09.00 h on day 2 after dexamethasone.

Long dexamethasone suppression test
Indications: A test to help differentiate the cause of Cushing's syndrome.
Note: DHAS estimations may be useful if a virilising tumour of the adrenal is suspected.
Assay request: serum cortisol.
Patient preparation: hospitalised.
Drug: Dexamethasone tablets 0·5 mg 6-hourly for 2 days, at 10.00 h (day 1), 16.00, 22.00 and 04.00 h, followed by dexamethasone tablets 2 mg 6-hourly for 2 days at 10.00, 16.00, 22.00 and 04.00 h.
Procedure: collect serum samples at 10.00 h on days 1, 3, 5.

TESTS OF PITUITARY FUNCTION

Indications: Diagnosis of diseases of hypothalamic/pituitary/gonadal/adrenal/thyroid axes.
1. Investigation of unexplained short stature with delay in bone age.
2. Investigation of other endocrine disorders including those of puberty which may be secondary to pituitary failure.
If there is unexplained short stature with delay in bone age proceed with screening tests detailed below. If screening tests positive or extreme short stature and growth hormone defi-

ciency is likely, estimate thyroxine (T_4) and if there is evidence of other trophic hormone deficiencies, check diurnal rhythm of serum cortisol. Then proceed to insulin sensitivity test.

Screening test for growth hormone deficiency.—The patient should fast from 18.00 h the previous evening or for a minumum of 12 h prior to the test. Blood is collected for blood glucose (1 ml in fluoride-oxalate tube) and for growth hormone estimation (plain tube, 2 ml to give 0·5 ml serum).

Glucose, 1·75 g/kg, but not more than 50 g, is then given orally, and further blood samples for glucose and growth hormone collected at 3, 4 and 5 h after the dose. At least one value for serum growth hormone should exceed 10 mU/l for an adequate response.

Insulin sensitivity test.—This test should be used to confirm growth hormone deficiency if suspected from the results of the screening test. A doctor should be in attendance throughout. The patient should fast from 18.00 h the previous evening or for a minimum of 12 h. A polythene cannula is inserted into an antecubital vein and a slow intravenous infusion of normal saline commenced 60 minutes before collection of samples. A three-way tap inserted between the cannula and infusion set allows blood samples to be taken without stress and dextrose or glucagon to be given if severe signs of hypoglycaemia occur. Soluble (crystalline, glucagon-free) insulin 0·1 unit/kg is given intravenously (0·05 unit/kg for children weighing less than 15 kg or with good evidence of panhypopituitarism). Blood is taken for blood glucose and serum cortisol at 0 min and at 30, 60, 90 and 120 min.

Time (minutes)	0	20	30	60	90	120
Assay for:						
Glucose	+	+	+	+	+	+
hGH	+		+	+	+	+
Cortisol	+		+	+	+	+
FSH	+		+	+		
LH	+		+	+		
TSH	+		+	+		
Prolactin	+					
Thyroxine	+					
Oestradiol (females) or						
Testosterone (males)	+					

If T_4 on initial test was low, follow insulin by TRH and estimate TSH according to the protocol. If the child is in the pubertal age range also test gonadal function by giving LHRH and include FSH and LH estimation. Additional FSH estimations at 30 and 60 min may be useful in disorders of puberty.

A fall in blood glucose by 50 per cent of the fasting value at 20–30 min is required for adequate stimulation of the pituitary adrenal axis. The blood glucose response (insulin sensitivity and hypoglycaemia unresponsiveness) considered alone is an unreliable indication of pituitary function (growth hormone and ACTH release) in childhood. Peak responses of growth hormone and cortisol occur at 60 min after insulin. A value exceeding 15 mU/l for growth hormone should be demonstrable at least once during the course of the test for an adequate response. The peak response of cortisol normally occurs at 60 min after insulin and should exceed 386 nmol/l.

Note: Blood samples for glucose (fluoride tubes) and serum thyroxine should be sent to the local laboratory. The endocrine laboratory will accept samples for the other hormone tests. Do *not* send serum for hGH assay unless glucose level falls to half of basal level or to less than 2·2 mmol/l. Glucose results should accompany request.

Drugs: Soluble (glucagon free) insulin 20 U/ml. Insulin I.V. 0·1 U/kg (usual) or 0·05 U/kg if suspected hypopituitarism with associated ACTH deficiency. Follow insulin immediately by 100 micrograms LHRH and 200 micrograms TRH I.V. and collect samples as tabulated.

THYROID FUNCTION TESTS

Not all of the new methods have yet been applied to the study of thyroid function in children of different ages and maturation. Normal values must therefore be regarded as tentative and related to the current methods available locally.

Serum Thyroxine (T_4)

Supersedes protein-bound iodide (PBI) and is the preferred *first* measurement when hypothyroidism or hyperthyroidism is suspected. Values are significantly but normally elevated in infancy. Thyroxine is low in primary hypothyroidism and decreased in malnutrition associated with hypoproteinaemia. Certain drugs may decrease T_4: indicate nature of drug when T_4 is requested.

Approximate basal reference values for children and adults:
60–135 nmol/l

Note: This data does not include values for infants.

Serum Tri-iodothyronine (T_3)

Regarded by some authorities as more biologically active than T_4. Radioimmunoassays of the desired specificity are available through Supraregional Assay Centres. This assay should only be requested when screening tests for hy*per*thyroidisim are equivocal.

Serum Thyroid Stimulating Hormone (TSH)

TSH is the pituitary trophic hormone regulating T_4 synthesis. Measurement of this hormone is important to confirm *primary* hypothyroidism when the serum T_4 is low. Basal TSH levels rise significantly in this condition. Note that basal levels are of little value when hypothyroidism *secondary* to pituitary TSH deficiency is suspected. In this situation the thyroid-releasing hormone (TRH) stimulation test is advocated (see below). For normal values see page 189.

Thyroid-releasing Hormone Stimulation Test (TRH or TRF test).

Indications: hypothyroidism secondary to pituitary TSH deficiency.

Assay request: Serum TSH.

Drug: TRH linear peptide 200 micrograms I.V.

Data for euthyroid children is sparse. In adults 50 per cent with pituitary disease have impaired responses. Substitution therapy in children should be based on other tests of thyroid function if an impaired response is obtained. There is considerable individual variation in normal responses from one euthyroid subject and another. As a guide to a normal response, 3–6 fold increase above basal levels can be expected. Patients with hypothalamic disorders of TRH production frequently show higher TSH values after TRH at 60 minutes, when compared to 30-minute samples.

Procedure.—The recumbent patient is given 200 micrograms of TRH as a single intravenous injection. Serum samples are taken before (0), and 30 and 60 minutes after the injection for TSH assay. Fasting unnecessary.

Serum Thyroxine-Binding Globulin (TBG)
Indication: High values are characteristic of hypothyroidism. Decreased values are found in hyperthyroidism. Indicated if low or high serum T_4 values are found with a normal serum TSH.

INVESTIGATION OF HYPOGLYCAEMIA

Severe, persistent hypoglycaemia in infancy or later childhood is uncommon but requires urgent investigation because of the likelihood of cerebral damage.
Diagnosis: The following broad categories should be considered:

Hepatic enzyme deficiencies
Hormone deficiencies
Hormone excess
Poisoning
Ketotic
Idiopathic.

If the diagnosis is suspected, check with Dextrostix and take blood for glucose level and insulin before demonstrating symptomatic relief from glucose administration. Unhaemolysed blood for insulin (see below) must be frozen as serum and stored at $-20°C$ for later investigation when a hypoglycaemic episode is suspected. The urine should be tested for ketones and for sugar by both a specific glucose oxidase method (Glucostix) and a non-specific method (Clinitest).

Hepatic enzyme deficiencies.—Hypoglycaemia may be due to enzyme defects in glycogen synthesis or degradation, gluconeogenesis or galactose or fructose metabolism. Hepatomegaly is usually present except in glycogen synthetase deficiency. The definitive diagnosis depends on the demonstration of enzyme deficiency in one or more tissues (see more detailed texts). A glucagon test (see Clayton *et al.*)[*] may be helpful.

* See page 189 for reference.

Hormone deficiencies.—Hypoglycaemia may occur in adrenal insufficiency due to primary hypoplasia or aplasia and in congenital adrenal hyperplasia when evidence of sodium loss or virilisation in females will also be present. Serum cortisol levels, together with Synacthen stimulation testing (see p. 192) should be performed. Serum 17-OH progesterone should be estimated if congenital adrenal hyperplasia is suspected. Symptomatic hypoglycaemia may arise in growth hormone deficiency due to a variety of pituitary/hypothalamic causes. In early infancy growth retardation may not be apparent. See page 194 for details of growth hormone estimation.

Hormone excess.—The most frequent and damaging cause of severe hypoglycaemia is hyperinsulinism. This may occur in association with beta cell nesidioblastosis, hyperplasia or adenoma formation and in the Weidemann-Beckwith syndrome. These conditions may all display leucine sensitive hypoglycaemia with symptoms occurring especially after cow's milk feeds. Definitive diagnosis depends on pancreatic histology. The diagnosis of excess insulin secretion is demonstrated by serum values taken during symptoms or by serial fasting specimens when inappropriately elevated serum insulin values may be found. Insulin values in excess of 10 mU/ml should be considered elevated when accompanied by blood glucose levels of 2·5 mmol/l or less. Stimulating tests using leucine, tolbutamide or glucagon are dangerous and are not required for confirmation of the diagnosis, although insulin levels may be performed during glucagon stimulation if the diagnosis is unclear.

Miscellaneous causes.—Alcohol, salicylates and unripe akee fruit ingestion may be associated with hypoglycaemia. Ketotic hypoglycaemia should be suspected in any child over one year of age with central nervous system symptoms and ketonuria, in the absence of hepatomegaly.

TESTS FOR INBORN ERRORS OF METABOLISM

Galactosaemia.—If on milk, a positive Benedict's (Clinitest) and negative glucose oxidase (Clinistix) is strongly suggestive. Do not exclude the diagnosis on this evidence. Confirm by erythrocyte enzyme assay.

Gangliosidoses.—GM_1–leucocyte β-galactosidase; GM_2–total leucocyte hexosaminidase and separation of isoenzymes A and B to distinguish infantile Tay-Sachs from the Sandhoff variant.

Glycogen storage diseases.—Glucagon test before and after carbohydrate feed (measure both glucose and lactate; see page 197), glucose during galactose infusion, and erythrocyte glycogen. Liver or leucocyte enzyme assay only for confirmation.

Homocystinuria.—Cyanide-nitroprusside test on urine. Plasma chromatography. Hypermethioninaemia especially in infancy. Treat prior to surgery or during dehydrating illness with pyridoxine 500 mg daily and reduce when the risk of thrombosis lessens.

Lesch-Nyhan syndrome.—Urine uric acid/creatinine ratio. Restrict dietary purine and pass urine directly into laboratory container or send in collecting bags: uric acid precipitates in normal ward container and may be lost.

Lipidaemias.—Plasma cholesterol, triglyceride and lipoprotein electrophoresis after a prolonged (18 h) fast.

Metachromatic leucodystrophy.—Leucocyte arysulphatase A.

Mucopolysaccharidoses.—24 h urine collection, kept cold, to avoid false reactions. Alcian Blue (not Toluidine Blue) spot test and bovine albumin (not CPC) turbidity test followed by electrophoresis of urinary MPS for typing.

Organic acidaemias.—Low standard bicarbonate (pH may be normal), gas chromatography of urine (kept frozen).

Phenylketonuria.—Plasma phenylalanine concentration.

Porphyria.—Quantitative urine aminolaevulinic acid (ALA) and porphobilinogen (PBG), copro- and uroporphyrin. Children in remission may require a glycine load before abnormal results can be demonstrated. Faecal porphyrins and erythrocyte protoporphyrin.

Suxamethonium sensitivity.—Plasma cholinesterase with and without dibucaine and fluoride inhibition. Urgent analysis is not necessary.

Wilson's disease.—Serum caeruloplasmin (phenylene diamine oxidase), urinary and plasma copper.

NOTE. Raine, D. N., *Treatment of Inherited Metabolic Disease*, 1975 (M. T. P., Lancaster) gives detailed advice on treating several diseases, and references reporting attempts to treat some 200 others, together with the sources of special dietary preparations throughout the world.

K.D.G.
P.H.W.R.
B.T.R.

X

PRIMARY CARE,
CASUALTY
AND
OUT-PATIENTS

COMMON SYMPTOMS SEEN IN CHILDREN'S OUT-PATIENTS OR CASUALTY

Many of the problems encountered are best treated by explanation and reassurance alone. In order to carry conviction with parents the doctor must listen to the history, carry out an appropriately full examination and any necessary investigation. The lay public in the U.K. has now matured beyond the need for placebo medication in most instances, provided they are satisfied that the doctor has done his job properly.

The official names of drugs are given except where none is available; doses of liquid preparations are given in mg. The "Usual Quantity" column is for guidance only but denotes a convenient and readily dispensable amount on F.P.10.

THE INFANT

Symptoms in infants	Points in diagnosis	TREATMENT General	TREATMENT Medicinal	Average dose at 6 months	Average dose at 1 year	Times/day	Usual quantity
Aphthous stomatitis	Ulceration, bleeding, pain and drooling. Lasts a week.	Reassure, ice cream. Avoid antibiotics.	Paracetamol paediatric elixir 120 mg/5 ml.	60 mg	120 mg	3	50 ml
			Bioral gel (carbenoxolone sodium 2%)	after meals			
Colic (three month)	Exclude infection, intussusception, torsion of testis. *Parental candidate for NAI.*	Listen, explain, sympathise and retain contact.	Dicyclomine elixir (Merbentyl) 10 mg/5 ml	5 mg		3	50 ml
Napkin rashes: (a) Ammoniacal	Odour, spares creases.	Expose to dry.	Benzalkonium 0·1% cream (Drapolene)	after each napkin change			25 g
			Hydrocortisone 1% and clioquinol 3% ointment			twice daily	25 g
(b) Thrush	Mouth patches. Satellite lesions around main rash.	Expose to dry.	Nystatin cream 100,000 U/g or miconazole nitrate 2% cream	after each napkin change			25 g 30 g
(c) Detergent	Clearly demarcated erythema.	Use soap flakes instead.	Zinc and castor oil ointment BPC	after each napkin change			25 g
Diarrhoea and vomiting	If clinically dehydrated, admit, see page 53. Exclude acute abdomen.	Boiled water+glucose (or sugar 1 teaspoon to 4 oz of water), also see page 117.	None. Avoid Lomotil. Kaolin of little value. Antibiotics not indicated, for exceptions see page 117.	"Home made" salt solutions are very risky			
Persistent vomiting	Check if thriving. If blood and mucus in vomit, for Ba. meal. Exclude chronic urinary disease.	Prop up, thicken feeds, reassure. Spontaneous remission by 1 year.	Infant Gaviscon (in severe cases) or thicken with Nestargel.	½–1 sachet with part of feed		3	10 sachets
							50 g
Blocked nose	Poor feeding, vomiting	Nasal toilet	Ephedrine 0·5% nose drops before feeds and sleep for one week.				10 ml
Croup	If drooling, dyspnoeic or toxic, admit.	Fluids. Humidify.	Amoxycillin suspension 125 mg/5 ml	62·5 mg	125 mg	3	100 ml
Cough, paroxysmal	Probably pertussis or bronchiolitis, see page 128	If infant at risk ?admit	Erythromycin paediatric mixture 125 mg/5 ml	125 mg	125 mg	4	100 ml

THE OLDER CHILD

Symptoms	Points in diagnosis	General	Medicinal	Average dose at 2 years	7 years	Times/day	Usual quantity
RESPIRATORY							
Cough	If productive	Simple postural drainage by mother.	Antibiotic appropriate to cough, swab or sputum.				
	If irritant		Pholcodine linctus BPC 5 mg/5 ml	2·5 ml	5 ml	3	100 ml
	If persistent X-ray sinuses. ? sinusitis.	Ensure proper use of nose drops.	Ephedrine 0·5% nose drops. 5 days.	frequently—at least 3-hourly in day			
Otitis media (pain in ear)	Inspect drum. Follow-up hearing.	Use analgesic, ephedrine nose drops 0·5%; avoid ear drops.	Under 5 years amoxycillin suspension 125 mg/5 ml	62·5 mg	125 mg	3	100 ml
			Over 5 years penicillin V tablets.	125 mg	250 mg	4	20 tabs
Wheeze (mild recurrent)	Usually asthma, very occasionally F.B.	Allergy search. X-ray once.	Ephedrine BPC elixir 15 mg/5 ml with promethazine elixir 5 mg/5 ml	15 mg	30 mg	3	100 ml
				10 ml	25 ml	3	100 ml
			Salbutamol (Ventolin) syrup 2 mg/5 ml	1 mg	2 mg	3	100 ml
GASTRO-INTESTINAL							
Spurious diarrhoea Encopresis Faecal retention	Careful history. P.R. essential. Rarely Hirschsprung's.	Listen, explain, reassure. Fluids, bran. May need treatment for 6–12 months in a paediatric clinic.	Sennoside (Senokot): syrup 7·5 mg/5 ml granules 15 mg/5 ml tabs. 7·5 mg	5 ml 5 ml —	5–10 ml 2–4 tabs.	once once once	100 ml 100 g. 50 tabs
			Lactulose (Duphalac) 3·35 mg/5 ml	5 ml	10 ml	3	300 ml
			Bisacodyl (Dulcolax) tabs. 5 mg.	—	5 mg	once	30 tabs
			Bisacodyl children's suppositories 5 mg	5 mg	5–10 mg	once	6
			Phosphate enema formula B BPC	50 ml	100 ml	once	—

GENITO-URINARY

Dysuria (and frequency) ± cloudy urine in girls	Exclude UTI (see below) and threadworms. Often vulvovaginitis. Look and swab.	Hygiene at toilet					
	Thrush unlikely	Hygiene at toilet	Dienoestrol cream 0·01% (sparingly to vestibule only)		Twice daily for one week only		78 g
	Thrush suspected	Hygiene at toilet	Nystatin cream 100,000 U/g or miconazole nitrate 2% cream		Twice daily for one week only		15 g 30 g
Nocturnal enuresis (over 5 years)	Exclude UTI (see below). Check emotional background. If daytime frequency as well ...	Listen, explain bladder drill.	Imipramine at night may be of temporary help.	—	25 mg		30 tabs
			Propantheline	—	15 mg	3	50 tabs
Proven urinary tract infection.	Often PUO only. Confirm on M.S.U. (preferably two). Use Dipslide or Uricult. Pure growth of 100,000 organisms/ml confirms. Protein and cells alone misleading.	Investigate proven cases and follow-up for one year.	Sulphadimidine for 1 week	250 mg	500 mg	4	30 tabs
			Co-trimoxazole mixture paediatric 240 mg/5 ml	5 ml	10 ml	2	100 ml
			tabs. paediatric 120 mg	2 tabs.	4 tabs.	2	100 tabs

GENERAL

Debility, lassitude and pallor (misdiagnosed as anaemia)	Exclude infection, rheumatoid, neoplasia, etc.	Supportive and sympathetic. If organic disease is unlikely, must be got back to school.	Only if specific cause found. No indication for iron or 'tonic'.				
Limb pains and nocturnal cramps.	Rarely rheumatoid, rheumatic or leukaemic. Affects legs only in active healthy child. Check Hb, WBC and diff. ESR.	Explanation and reassurance.	Some relief from rubbing. Paracetamol if severe.		500 mg	once	30 tabs.

B.S.B.W.

FITS IN CHILDHOOD

Fits in childhood and their treatment may be grouped as follows:

1. *Neonatal fits.*—These are often symptomatic of a treatable condition. Diazepam may be used and phenobarbitone can be helpful.
2. *Infantile spasms* (West's syndrome).—Corticosteroids or ACTH are useful to begin with, then nitrazepam, clonazepam or sodium valproate should be used for long-term control, which is often difficult.
3. *Febrile convulsions.*—Intravenous diazepam is the drug of choice in controlling convulsions. Arguments over prophylaxis continue—sodium valproate may be preferable to phenobarbitone.
4. *Myoclonic astatic epilepsy* (Lennox syndrome).—Sodium valproate, nitrazepam and clonazepam are preferred for maintenance therapy. Where there is evidence of photosensitivity sodium valproate is the drug of choice.
5. *Petit mal* (absences).—With 3 c/s spike and wave, this responds to sodium valproate and at times to ethosuximide. When the absences are associated with automatisms sodium valproate is indicated.
6. *Grand mal* (tonic clonic seizures).—Sodium valproate is the drug of choice—it does not sedate and the incidence of side-effects is low. Phenytoin can be used but it has undesirable side-effects in females and serum levels are required to monitor dosage.
7. *Focal fits* (motor or sensory).—Respond best to carbamazepine: sensory fits may be difficult to control—phenobarbitone, primidone or phenytoin may be helpful.
8. *Temporal lobe epilepsy* (psychomotor fits).—Carbamazepine is the preferred drug. Phenytoin can be helpful.

Once fits are controlled sodium valproate, phenobarbitone, phenytoin and ethosuximide can be given once a day, preferably in the evenings. Carbamazepine has to be given twice, and occasionally three, times a day. The table summarises starting dose, therapeutic range and side-effects.

ANTICONVULSANTS

Drug	Individual Starting Dose		Times per 24 h	Therapeutic Range		Side-Effects	
	Average child	mg/kg		µg/ml	µmol/l	Minor (often dose related)	Major (usually uncommon)
Carbamazepine Tabs 100, 200 mg Syrup 100 mg/5 ml	200–400 mg (N.B. gradual dose increments)	10	2	4–10	16–50	Lethargy, dizziness (if dose increased too rapidly). Dry mouth, G.I. disturbance, diplopia	Purpura, blood dyscrasia, jaundice (v. rare). Inappropriate ADH secretion
Clonazepam Tabs 0.5, 2 mg	0.25–0.5 mg	0.1–0.2	1	—	—	Sedation, hypotonia, drooling	Bronchial hypersecretion, ataxia
Ethosuximide Caps 250 mg Syrup 250 mg/5 ml	250–500 mg	15–25	2	40–100	280–700	Sedation, ataxia, G.I. disturbance	Blood dyscrasias
Nitrazepam Tabs/caps 5 mg	2.5–5.0 mg	0.5–1.0	1	—	—	Sedation, drooling	Bronchial hypersecretion
Phenytoin Tab 25, 50, 100 mg Cap 25, 50, 100 mg Infatabs 50 mg Susp. 30 mg/5 ml	50–100 mg (N.B. gradual dose increments)	5	2	5–20	20–100	Rash, G.I. disturbance, sedation, ataxia, gum hypertrophy. Hirsutism, acne and coarsening of features in adolescent girls	Nystagmus, blood dyscrasia
Phenobarbitone Tab 15, 30, 60 mg	15–30 mg	3	2	15–30	40–105	Sedation. May cause hyper-excitability in a few children	May impair learning ability. Vertigo, headache, nausea
Sodium valproate Tab 200, 500 mg (Also E/C) Syrup 200 mg/5 ml	200–400 mg	20–50	2 (1)	No established range		G.I. disturbances, transient hair loss, tremor	Bleeding, thrombocytopenia. Liver dysfunction rare

GENETIC INVESTIGATION AND COUNSELLING

The Indications for Chromosomal Analysis

(a) Sexual ambiguity, including cryptorchidism.
(b) Unexplained short stature in a girl.
(c) Primary amenorrhoea.
(d) Sexual infantilism.
(e) Unexplained mental retardation (particularly if associated with malformation such as cleft palate, coloboma of eye, congenital heart defect, deformity of ears, defects of hands and feet).
(f) Infants suspected of having trisomy 21, 18 or 13.*
(g) Other newborn infants with multiple defects (as listed in (e)).

GENETIC COUNSELLING

The recurrence risk of disorders will frequently be of interest to parents; when it is very low, as is usual in mongolism or most rare malformations, or very high, as in fibrocystic disease, the parents should normally be informed.

Simple genetic disorders in man are due either to mutations which may be recent and unlikely to recur in sibs born to normal parents (e.g. in trisomy 21 or a dominant disorder such as achondroplasia) or they may be due to some distant mutation as in almost all cases of autosomal recessive disorders (e.g. albinism, fibrocystic disease) and many cases of sex-linked disorder (e.g. haemophilia, Duchenne's dystrophy).

* Most correctly diagnosed cases have an extra free-lying chromosome. In a few infants the extra chromosome material is found to be translocated onto another chromosome; in such cases the chromosomes of both parents must always be analysed. As these are often normal it must be assumed that the translocation was a recent and isolated event and therefore unlikely to recur, but sometimes one or other parent has a balanced arrangement and therefore runs the risk of having further affected infants. For example 6 per cent of mongols have a 21 translocation but only a third of these have a parent with a balanced translocation. Trisomy 21 may recur in a sibship if the mother is a mongol or mongol mosaic (trisomy 21/normal). A number of apparently normal mothers have been discovered with this form of mosaicism which can only be excluded by careful chromosomal analysis. The incidence of trisomy 21 depends on maternal age. Below 30 years the risk is 1–2000. At about 35 years the incidence is 1–500; at 38 years, 1–180; at 40 years, 1–100; at 45 years, 1–50.

In congenital malformations, as in all diseases, there is a familial tendency but this is usually too small to influence further conceptions. In almost all malformations the aetiology is unknown and the empiric recurrence risk is 3 to 5 per cent, and about 10 per cent after two affected children.

In recessively determined disorders in which the diagnosis is accurate, and legitimacy can be assumed, the recurrence risk is 25 per cent. The commonest forms include fibrocystic disease, albinism, the adrenogenital syndrome, and haemoglobinopathies.

In sex-linked disorders, such as haemophilia and Duchenne's muscular dystrophy, isolated cases may be due to either new or old mutants and there may, or may not, be increased risk.

Dominant conditions, such as the common form of achondroplasia, are rare and, if the parents are free of disease and the diagnosis accurate, it may be assumed that this is due to a new mutation carrying no realistic risk of recurrence.

AMNIOCENTESIS

Selective abortion is feasible when the diagnosis can be made from the examination of supernatant amniotic fluid or by examining amniotic fluid cells in cases where the defect is expressed in these cells.

At present alpha-fetoprotein is the main constituent routinely sought in supernatant fluid. The level is raised whenever the protein has the opportunity to leak out from the fetus as in open neural tube defects, some cases of exomphalos, congenital nephrosis and fetal death. Cells can be examined for nuclear sex bodies, chromosomes and certain rare and specific metabolic disorders.

The main indications for sixteen-week amniocentesis are:

Chromosomal
1. When a parent has a balanced translocation or rearrangement.
2. Mother has had a previous trisomic mongol.
3. Maternal age over 38 years.

Alpha-fetoprotein (for open neural tube defect)
1. Previous neural tube defect baby.
2. Parental spina bifida.
3. High maternal serum AFP taken after 16th week of a singleton pregnancy.

Sex chromatin
X-linked disease if mother probably a carrier.

Metabolic Disease

Few laboratories are competent to culture and test for those rare metabolic disorders amenable to antenatal diagnosis. Clinical genetics and paediatric biochemical departments hold current lists of conditions that are recognisable and the laboratories willing to advise on and undertake the tests.

A precise antenatal diagnosis may not always be easily achieved. Much depends on the accuracy of the biochemical diagnosis in the propositus and the experience of the laboratory. It is good policy to check the biochemical diagnosis in the propositus with the laboratory that may later be asked to perform antenatal diagnosis on the prospective sibling (or male relative in X-linked disease). A timely skin biopsy taken from the propositus, cultured and then stored in liquid nitrogen, ensures that tissue for biochemical comparison is still available after the death of the propositus.

Carrier detection is available for a number of diseases. In haemophilia the prediction depends on estimates of factor VIII and factor VIII related antigen, with each laboratory determining its norms. Carrier detection is also available for Duchenne muscular dystrophy using creatine phosphokinase estimation and pedigree data. Unfortunately (as with many enzyme estimations) results vary even between laboratories using the same technique. As one-third of obligative carriers have results within the normal range, and prediction depends on the mean level of three samples, estimations should only be made in designated laboratories whose C.P.K. values have been evaluated by extensive family studies. The clinical genetic service will answer queries about carrier detection as well as those relating to antenatal diagnosis.

Fetoscopy

The fetus can be examined through a fibre-optic instrument introduced after ultrasound localisation. Individual parts may be viewed and fetal blood sampled, but the procedure is not without risk and even in the best hands this includes a 3 per cent risk of accidental fetal death.

J.I.

MANAGEMENT OF CHILDREN WITH NON-ACCIDENTAL INJURIES ("BATTERED BABY" SYNDROME)

The diagnosis of child abuse is often missed, and trauma inflicted by the parents must be considered in any case where symptoms remain unexplained. These children often present to the Casualty Department, and the diagnosis should be suspected in any young child presenting with bruising, particularly of the face, and/or with underlying fractures.

Diagnosis

History.—Suspicion should be aroused when:
(a) There has been delay in taking the child to a doctor.
(b) There is inadequate, discrepant or excessively plausible explanation of the injury.
(c) The child or a sibling has previously attended hospital with an injury, or when a history of previous injury is obtained.
(d) There is evidence of repeated injury or of the co-existence of different types of injury, e.g. burns, fractures, bruises.
(e) The child is frequently brought to the doctor or hospital for little apparent reason.
(f) Parents exhibit disturbed behaviour or unusual reaction to the child's injuries.
(g) The child fails to thrive or shows obvious neglect.

Examination.—At first sight the injuries may appear trivial, for example: small facial bruises, burns or abrasions; injuries to the mouth; injuries caused by severe shaking, e.g. bruising from handling. A full examination of the child is essential to detect any other new or old injuries, followed by a skeletal survey.

Immediate Management

If the diagnosis seems at all possible
1. *Admit the child* to hospital. This should be done whether or not the actual medical and surgical findings are severe enough to warrant admission. Admission offers an opportunity to assess and protect the child and to gather information on the dynamics of the family.

2. *Record carefully* the history and clinical findings with diagrams and measurements.
3. *Skeletal survey* (X-ray of long bones, ribs and skull) is essential and consultation with the radiologist will be most helpful in estimating the date of any fractures.
4. *Exclude a bleeding disorder* both for medical and legal reasons.
5. *Photographs* (black and white and coloured) are helpful in documenting findings.
6. *Check out attendances of child and siblings* at local hospitals (especially for injury).
7. Arrange to *examine siblings* at this stage if diagnosis seems certain.
8. Liaise with G.P. and Health Visitor.
9. *Ward Staff and Senior Nursing Staff must be clearly informed:*
   (*a*) of reason for admission,
   (*b*) whether on a "voluntary" basis by consent of parent(s) or on a compulsory basis (Place of Safety Order already obtained or being sought),
   (*c*) which member of the medical staff to contact if trouble arises.
10. *No accusations* should be made against the parents as this antagonises them and makes further management complicated.
11. *Refer the parents to a Medical Social Worker* for further family investigation.
12. *The paediatrician-in-charge should make the decision about involving the police or social services:* when a Medical Social Worker is involved this will be in consultation.

Chain of Identification

As information may subsequently be required for evidence in Court, it is important for medical staff to establish a careful, unbroken *chain of identification* between the patient and other medical and paramedical staff involved in that patient's investigations (such as blood tests, photographs and X-rays). Samples of blood and body fluids and request forms should all be carefully and clearly labelled and bear a legible signature. On the request form it should also be clearly recorded (1) who performed the venepuncture, (2) who transported the sample to the laboratory (ideally (1) and (2) should be the same person),and (3) who received the samples in the laboratory. The child should be formally identified to the Medical Photographer who should be clearly shown the injuries to be recorded. Without this meticulous attention to detail, loopholes may be found in evidence and efforts aimed at protecting the child from further risk may be rendered invalid.

Subsequent Management

Discussion with the parents should be the responsibility of an experienced paediatrician, who will assess the mental status of the parents and make recommendations on the subsequent management of the family. Although every effort will be made to maintain the family unit the child's safety is the aim of management. It may be necessary to bring the child before the Juvenile Court so that on discharge from hospital its safety may be safeguarded.

The house physician may be confronted by an irate parent demanding the discharge of his child. Every effort should be made to placate such parents and to explain that the child's medical condition is still under investigation. If despite such effort the parents insist on discharge, the action recommended is:

1. Contact the registrar or consultant in charge of the case and inform them that the parents are insisting on discharging their child against medical advice.
2. If the consultant feels that it is not in the child's interests to be discharged at the present time, the Social Services Department should be contacted. An application will be made by this department to the Justice of the Peace who can order that the child remains in hospital.
3. If for any reason there is a delay or difficulty in obtaining a safety order, the Police Department should be contacted by a member of the medical staff.

M.A.T.

REPORTING DEATHS TO THE CORONER

In deaths in the following circumstances the doctor is advised to inform the coroner as soon as possible:

All Deaths which are sudden or unexpected and where the Doctor cannot certify the real, as opposed to the terminal, cause of death or where the Doctor has not attended in the last illness or within fourteen days of death.

Abortions—other than natural.

Accidents and Injuries of any date, if in any way contributing to the cause of death.

Alcoholism—chronic or acute.

Anaesthetics and Operations—deaths while under the influence of anaesthetics and deaths following operation for injury or where the operation, however necessarily or skilfully performed, may have precipitated or expedited death.

Crime or Suspected Crime.

Drugs—therapeutic mishaps, abuse or addiction.

Ill-Treatment—starvation or neglect.

Industrial Diseases arising out of the deceased's employment, e.g. pneumoconiosis, Weil's disease and all diseases and poisons covered by the Factories Acts.

Infant Deaths—if in any way obscure.

Pensioners receiving Disability Pensions. Where death might be connected with the pensionable disability.

Persons in Legal Custody—in a Prison, Borstal Institution or Approved School, or any Detention Quarters even if the death was in hospital.

Persons suffering from mental disorders are to be reported only if they fall into one of the general categories.

Poisoning from any cause, occupational, therapeutic, accidental, suicidal, homicidal; also food poisoning.

Septicaemias—if originating from an injury or an operation.

Stillbirths—where there may be a possibility of the child having been born alive, or where there is suspicion.

N.B. A provisionally registered practitioner can only sign a death certificate in the course of his duties at an approved institution.

Cremation Certificate Form C can only be signed by a practitioner who has been fully registered for more than five years (any period of provisional registration does not qualify).

Apart from the general rule of law some Coroners have special wishes, such as requesting that deaths within 24 hours of admission should be reported to him.

Sudden infant death syndrome (cot deaths) would automatically be reported and any case where there has been recent or possibly relevant injury should also be reported. The reasons for this are not bureaucratic formality but to avoid inconvenience and distress to relatives if the death certificate is questioned at the Registrar's office and possibly reported to the Coroner at this stage. If in doubt therefore it is best to ring the Coroner's Officer and this will smooth the passage of the certificate and does not necessarily result in a post-mortem.

Advice on Attending an Inquest

First, it is important to attend the post-mortem with all the relevant clinical notes and X-rays. If required to attend the inquest, the doctor should be punctual, bring the relevant documents and refresh his memory from the notes and statements on the evidence, especially regarding dates, times and special procedures. The medical evidence will help to achieve the objects of an inquest which are:

1. To ascertain on behalf of the Crown whether any criminal act was relevant, but equally important are the following:
2. To bring out all the evidence about what happened so that the relatives will have as complete a picture as possible as to how death occurred; this may prevent subsequent criticism of medical treatment given.
3. To try to see if anything can be learnt or done with a view to preventing similar tragedies.
4. To reach a verdict.

USEFUL ADDRESSES FOR FAMILIES AND THEIR DOCTORS

Arthritis and Rheumatism
  Council
Faraday House
8–10 Charing Cross Road
London WC2H 0HN
Tel. (01) 240 0871

British Diabetic Association
10 Queen Anne Street
London W1M 0BD
Tel. (01) 323 1531

British Epilepsy Association
Crowthorne House
New Wokingham Road
Wokingham, Berks. RG11
  3AY
Tel. Wokingham 3122

British Institute for the
  Mentally Handicapped
Wolverhampton Road
Kidderminster, Worcs.
  DY10 3PP
Tel. Kidderminster 850251

British Kidney Patients
  Association
Bordon, Hants.
Tel. Bordon 2022

British Migraine
  Association
178a High Road
Byfleet, Weybridge
Surrey, KT14 7ED
Tel. Byfleet 52468

Brittle Bones Association
63 Byron Crescent
Dundee, DD3 6SS
Tel. Dundee 827130

Coeliac Society
P.O. Box 181
London NW2 2QY
Tel. (01) 459 2440

Chest, Heart and Stroke
  Association
Tavistock Square North
Tavistock Square
London WC1H 9JE
Tel. (01) 387 3012

The Compassionate Friends
(support for bereaved
  parents)
7 Paulsdene Crescent
Salisbury, Wilts
Tel. Salisbury 27774

Cystic Fibrosis Research
  Trust
5 Blyth Road
Bromley, Kent BR1 3RS
Tel. (01) 464 7211

Down's Children's
  Association
Quinborne Community
  Centre
Ridgacre Road
Birmingham, B32 2TW
Tel. Birmingham 427 1374

The Family Fund (for
  families of severely
  handicapped children)
P.O. Box 50
York, YO1 1UY

Foundation for the Study of
  Infant Deaths (cot deaths)
4 Grosvenor Place
London SW1X 7HD
Tel. (01) 235 1721

GINGERBREAD
  (Association of one-
  parent families)
35 Wellington Street
London WC2
Tel. (01) 240 0953

Haemophilia Society
16 Trinity Street
London SE1 1DE
Tel. (01) 407 1010

Lady Hoare Trust for
  Physically Handicapped
  Children
7 North Street
Midhurst
West Sussex, GU29 9DJ
Tel. Midhurst 081 3696

Leukaemia Society
Hamlyns View
St. Andrews Road
Exeter, Devon

Malcolm Sargent Cancer
  Fund for Children
6 Sydney Street
London SW3 6PP
Tel. (01) 352 6884

Muscular Dystrophy Group
  of Great Britain
35 Macaulay Road
London SW4 0QP
Tel. (01) 720 8055

National Association of
  Deaf Blind and Rubella
  Handicapped
86 Cleveland Road
Ealing, London W13
Tel. (01) 991 0513

National Association for
  Spina Bifida and
  Hydrocephalus
Tavistock House North
Tavistock Square
London WC1H 9HJ
Tel. (01) 388 1382

National Association for the
  Welfare of Children in
  Hospital
7 Exton Street
London SE1 8VE
Tel. (01) 261 1738

National Deaf Children's
  Society
45 Hereford Road
London W2 5AH
Tel. (01) 229 9272

National Society for Autistic
  Children
1a Golders Green Road
London NW11 8EA
Tel. (01) 458 4375

National Society for
  Epileptics
Chalfont St. Peter
Bucks, SL9 0RJ
Tel. Chalfont St. Giles 3991

National Society for
  Mentally Handicapped
  Children
117–123 Golden Lane
London EC1Y 0RT
Tel. (01) 253 9433

Royal National Institute for
  the Blind
224 Great Portland Street
London W1N 6AA
Tel. (01) 388 1266

Royal National Institute for
  the Deaf
105 Gower Street
London WC1E 6AH
Tel. (01) 387 8033

Safety in Playgrounds
  Action Group
85 Dalston Drive
Manchester, M2O 0LQ

Spastics Society
12 Park Crescent
London W1N 4EQ
Tel. (01) 580 3226

Stillbirth and Perinatal
  Death Association
15a Christchurch Hill
London NW3 1JY
Tel. (01) 794 4601

Toy Libraries Association
Wyllyotts Manor
Darkes Lane
Potters Bar, EN6 5HL
Tel. Potters Bar 44571

Tuberous Sclerosis
  Association of Great
  Britain
Church Farm House
Church Road
North Leigh
Oxford, OX8 6TX
Tel. Oxford 881238

Voluntary Council for
  Handicapped Children
(National Children's
  Bureau)
8 Wakley Street
London EC1V 7QE
Tel. (01) 278 9441

[NOTES]

[NOTES]

[NOTES]

[NOTES]

[NOTES]

[NOTES]

[NOTES]

XI
PAEDIATRIC PRESCRIBING

NOTES FOR PRESCRIBERS

All preparations should be written clearly using approved abbreviations. In general, single drugs should be prescribed using the approved name wherever possible. The name of the drug should be printed in block letters. Metric doses must be used and whenever possible decimal points should be eliminated. The approved abbreviation of gramme is "g" and of milligramme is "mg". Micrograms should be written in full. Except for compound formulations, substitutes for dose weights, e.g. Caps, Tabs, Vials, etc., must be avoided.

Abbreviations such as "P.R.N." and "S.O.S." should not be used. The symptom or sign to be relieved must be written in prescribing instructions of this nature and the maximum frequency of administration should be clearly stated, e.g. "As required for headache—maximum 4-hourly". Only the following routes of administration should be abbreviated:

Intravenous—I.V.	Inhalation—INHAL.
Intramuscular—I.M.	Per rectum—P.R.
Intrathecal—I.T.	Subcutaneous—S.C.
Intradermal—I.D.	Topical—TOP.

"Oral" and other routes of administration should be written in full for each prescription.

For oral liquid preparations, wherever possible the dose is supplied in a 5 ml volume and the patient issued with a 5 ml spoon. However, reasons of stability and palatability sometimes dictate a different dose volume; it is better for the prescriber to order the required dose, leaving the volume to the pharmacist.

The labels of all dispensed preparations should bear full details of content unless otherwise requested.

Prescriptions for Controlled Drugs must state dose, total number of doses written in both figures and letters, frequency of administration of the drug, bear the full signature (initials are not sufficient) of a registered Medical/Dental Practitioner and the date. Obviously the name of the patient, registration number and address, where applicable, should be stated.

The full signature of the prescriber should be used when each prescription is written for any drug and when discontinuing treatment. A choice of route, e.g. oral/I.V./I.M., should never be written; a complete prescription is required for each route. Similarly no amendment to dose or frequency should be made without a new prescription being written.

Rational prescribing may be defined as "the prescribing of drugs that are safe and efficacious, while taking into account current knowledge of drug action, the needs of the patient and costs".

Having decided to use a certain drug, it is necessary to consider the best method of achieving the objective of therapy—effective concentration of drug at the expected site of action as quickly and conveniently as possible for the patient.

Route and Preparation

Oral—for ease and convenience liquid preparations are generally more acceptable for children under 5 years as well as for some older ones. In order to reduce dental caries and gingivitis in children requiring long-term medication, non-sucrose containing liquids are preferred. It is possible for even young patients to be given crushed tablets if the required strength is available.

Parenteral—intravenous administration is generally least painful and most appropriate, especially if peripheral perfusion is poor.

Rectal—cannot be relied upon to produce adequate blood levels of drugs. It should probably be reserved for diazepam (and perhaps paraldehyde) administration when attempting to stop a convulsion in the home or for controlling sickness due to cytotoxic therapy.

Topical—has limited therapeutic possibilities, but is indicated for certain skin conditions.

N.B. Absorption of topical steroid preparations is enhanced in infants and young children and poorly controlled therapy with potent steroids can cause growth retardation and adrenal insufficiency. The minimum concentration of steroid to achieve clinical improvement should be prescribed using either a commercially available preparation of low potency or a suitable dilution of a stronger one.

Dose Size

Many formulae have been devised to aid dosage calculation for children. Most involve fractioning of adult doses based on age or weight and are not accurate for all children. Relating dosage to body surface is perhaps most useful but this also fails to take into account the differences between children and adults in some pharmacokinetic parameters and tissue responsiveness.

It is believed that the following dosage tables apply to a comprehensive range of drugs. If clinicians wish to prescribe drugs which are not included in these tables, it is suggested that all available drug information and literature sources be consulted.

Difficulties will arise when the lack of appropriate dose size formulations prevents accurate dose calculations. The clinician must then use his own judgment.

Doses may need adjustment because of renal or hepatic insufficiency, fever or gastro-intestinal disease. Refer to a reputable text.

Dose and Frequency

Because children in general metabolise drugs more quickly than adults, doses may need to be given more frequently to maintain an effective drug level. It may be necessary to give a loading dose as the rate of metabolism of the drug affects the time taken to reach the steady state. Unless a loading dose is used the time to reach this steady state will be at least 5 times the half-life of the drug, regardless of how often the drug is given.

N.B. (a) For both size and frequency, the figures given in the tables are based on a combination of reduction of adult weight-related dose, clinical studies in children and empirical use.

(b) Doses in the columns refer to single doses and when continuing therapy is required, the recommended number of times per 24 hours is shown in column three.

Once the dose has been calculated, prescribers should refer to the right-hand column of the dosage section for a guide to preparations available.

Drug Level Monitoring

It is particularly important to monitor drug levels in children because of the greater inter- and intra-individual variation in drug response in this age range than at any other time in life.

Unfortunately few therapeutic ranges have been reported specifically in children and extrapolation from adult data is not wholly appropriate. The comments section therefore only includes levels for those drugs in which a paediatric therapeutic range has been established.

Adverse Effects

These are often unrecognised and under-reported in children, particularly in the newborn. All reactions to recently introduced drugs and serious or unusual reactions to other drugs should be reported to the Committee on Safety of Medicines. It is suggested that parents should be informed of the likely effects of drugs, especially those which may cause discomfort, and so hope to avoid poor compliance. The most frequently observed reactions in infants and children are shown in Table XVI.

Drug Interactions

Most drug interactions are of greater theoretical interest than of practical importance. In the clinical situation, enzyme inducing agents, e.g. carbamazepine, phenobarbitone, phenytoin and rifampicin, tend to decrease the effect of important drugs with hepatic metabolism, e.g. each other, chloramphenicol, isoniazid and steroids. Enzyme inhibitors, e.g. chloramphenicol, diazepam, isoniazid and sodium valproate, sometimes increase the effects of drugs metabolised by the hepatic microsomal enzyme system, e.g. most anticonvulsant agents. Aspirin and sodium valproate may displace phenytoin from its protein binding sites, increasing its effect. For more detailed information on drug interactions consult your pharmacist.

I.V. Incompatibilities

If two drugs have to be combined for I.V. therapy then consult your pharmacist for a chart of incompatibilities before the drugs are mixed. In general, few drugs are compatible, e.g. ampicillin and flucloxacillin are compatible; gentamicin and flucloxacillin are not.

TABLE XVI

The most frequently observed drug reactions and the likely cause
in infants and children outside the newborn period.

System	Effect	Drug
Gastro-intestinal	Nausea and vomiting Diarrhoea } Monilial infection }	Most drugs See page 255
Haematological	Bone marrow suppression Megaloblastic anaemia	Chloramphenicol Cytotoxics Phenytoin Co-trimoxazole
Cutaneous	Macular and/or papular rash Urticaria Alopecia	Ampicillin Phenytoin Penicillins Sodium valproate Cytotoxics
Neurological	Drowsiness Ataxia Dyskinesia Hyperkinesis	Phenobarbitone Carbamazepine Phenytoin Carbamazepine Metoclopramide Prochlorperazine Phenobarbitone
Metabolic	Hypokalaemia Hyperglycaemia Cushingoid syndrome Short stature	Frusemide Prednisolone Thiazides Corticosteroids Cortocosteroids (long- term)
Cardiovascular	Bradycardia Hypertension	Digoxin Prednisolone

[NOTES]

SOME IMPORTANT DRUGS

Drug	Route	Times Daily	DOSE Caution. Suggested dose is single dose unless otherwise stated					Availability and Remarks
			0-2/52 Neonatal	2/52-1 year	1 year	7 years	14 plus	
Acetazolamide	Oral	Once	—	—	125 mg	250 mg	500 mg	Tab. 250 mg scored. Sustets 500 mg. Twice daily for glaucoma
Adrenaline inj. 1-1000	S.C.	Single dose	0·01 ml/kg		0·12 ml	0·25 ml	0·5 ml	
Allopurinol	Oral	3	—	5 mg/kg	50 mg	100 mg	200 mg	Prevention of uric acid nephropathy. N.B. Potentiates 6-Mercaptopurine—reduce 6MP dose by 75%. See page 171. Tabs. 100 mg.
Aluminium hydroxide mixture B.P.C.	Oral	3 or 4	—	—	1 ml / 5 ml	2·5 ml / 10-20 ml	5 ml	Dose for phosphate binding in renal disease. Antacid dose.
Aminocaproic acid (E.A.C.A.)	Oral	4	—	100 mg/kg	1·5 g	3 g	6 g	Eff. Powder and Syrup. Management of oral bleeding in coagulation disorders. See also Tranexamic Acid.
Aminophylline	See under Theophylline, page 245							
Amitriptyline HCl	Oral	3	—	—	—	10 mg	25 mg	Antidepressant dose—may be doubled.
		ONCE at night	—	—	—	10 mg-25 mg may need 50-75 mg		Nocturnal enuresis dose. Tab. 10 mg and 25 mg. Syrup.
Asparaginase	I.V.	For Leukaemia see page 172.						Warning: may cause anaphylaxis
Aspirin and soluble aspirin	Oral	3 or 4	Suggest Paracetamol			300 mg	600 mg	Antipyretic/analgesic dose. Tabs. and Soluble Tabs. 300 mg.
		4-6	—		50-75 mg/kg/24 hours.			Anti-inflammatory dose. Adjust to Salicylate level of 1000-2000 micromoles/l.

SOME IMPORTANT DRUGS—*(continued)*

Drug	Route	Times Daily	DOSE. Caution. Suggested dose is single dose unless otherwise stated					Availability and Remarks
			0–2/52 Neonatal	2/52–1 year	1 year	7 years	14 plus	
Atropine methonitrate	Oral	Before feeds	50 microg/kg				—	"Eumydrin". Drops only.
Atropine sulphate	Oral or S.C.	Single	15 microg/kg		150 microg	300 microg	600 microg	Tabs. 600 microg. Pre-op. dose.
Bendrofluazide	Oral	Once	1·25 mg		1·25 mg	2·5 mg	5 mg	Tabs. 2·5 mg, 5 mg. K^+ supplements may be required, see page 56.
Benorylate	Oral	4		—	15–30 mg/kg		2 g	Tab. 750 mg. Susp. For Rheumatoid arthritis.
Bephenium hydroxynaphthoate	Oral		See page 262					Sachets 5 g. Hookworms (*Ancylostomiasis*) and Roundworms (*Ascariasis*).
Calciferol (Vit. D_2)	Oral	Once	3000 units to 5000 units					Calciferol-sensitive rickets dose. Tabs. 3000 and 50,000 units.
Calcium chloride as dihydrate	Oral	4	33 mg/kg		330 mg		—	See page 154. 5 ml Inj. $CaCl_2$. $2H_2O$ contains 2·5 mmol Ca^{++} = 100 mg Ca^{++} (0·45 ml = 33 mg $CaCl_2$. $2H_2O$).
Calcium gluconate	Oral	4	100 mg/kg		1 g	2 g	4 g	1 g = 2·25 mmol Ca^{++} = 90 mg Ca^{++}. See pages 81, 91. Tabs. 300 mg and 600 mg. Syrup. Effervescent Tabs. 1 g. Caution—Bradycardia.
	I.V.	Single	See p. 91	30 mg/kg Slow I.V. using 10% Inj. diluted to 2·5% solution.				
Carbamazepine	Oral	2 or 3	—	10–20 mg/kg	100 mg	200 mg	400 mg	Anticonvulsant dose. Tabs. 100 mg and 200 mg.
Carbimazole	Oral	3	0·25 mg/kg		2·5 mg	5mg	10 mg	Initial dose stated. Reduce total daily dose to 1/3 or 1/4 when symptoms controlled and give as single daily dose. Tabs. 5 mg.

Drug	Route	Doses					Notes
Chloral hydrate	Oral	3	30 mg/kg				Single hypnotic dose can be doubled.
Chlorpheniramine	Oral / S.C. or I.V.	3 or 4 / Single	— / 0·25 mg/kg	1 mg / 2·5 mg	2 mg / 5 mg	4 mg / 10 mg	Dose may be safely doubled. Tabs. 4 mg and Syrup. Sustained-release 8 mg and 12 mg.
Chlorpromazine	Oral or I.M.	3 or 4	1 mg/kg	10 mg	25 mg	50 mg	Sedative/Antiemetic dose stated. Psychiatric dose—stated dose × 2. Tabs. 10 mg, 25 mg, 50 mg and 100 mg. Syrup.
Choline theophyllinate			See under Theophylline, page 245.				
Cimetidine	Oral / I.V.	4	—	5–10 mg/kg		200 mg	Tab. 200 mg. Syrup and Inj. Adjust dose in renal impairment.
Clonazepam	Oral maint. / I.V.	2 / Single dose	— / —	500 microg / 50 microg/kg slowly	1 mg /	2 mg / 30–40 microg/kg slowly	4 mg / 25 microg/kg slowly → Tab. 500 microg and 2 mg. May cause drowsiness, start with lower doses inc. to maint. Dose for status epilepticus. Titrate according to response. Caution—transient respiratory depression.
Cyclophosphamide	Oral / I.V.	Once / Once	—	For use in Leukaemia and neoplasms see page 172.		3 mg/kg	Dose for nephrotic syndrome where indicated. Tab. 10 mg and 50 mg.
Cytosine arabinoside	I.V. / S.C.	Once	For use in Leukaemia see page 172.				For I/T do NOT use special diluent.
Daunorubicin	I.V.	Once	For use in Leukaemia see page 172.				Total cumulative dose not to exceed 350 mg/m² because of cardiotoxicity.
Desferrioxamine mesylate			In iron-poisoning, see page 153.				Seek advice for chelation in transfusion dependent patients. See page 166.
Desmopressin (DDAVP)	Nasal / I.M. / I.V.	1 or 2 / Single	— / —		5–10 microg / 400 nanog	10–20 microg / 1–4 microg	Nasal soln. 100 microg/ml. For diabetes insipidus.

SOME IMPORTANT DRUGS—(continued)

Drug	Route	Times Daily	DOSE Caution. Suggested dose is single dose unless otherwise stated					Availability and Remarks
			0-2/52 Neonatal	2/52- 1 year	1 year	7 years	14 plus	
Diazepam	Oral	2	—	50 microg/kg	500 microg	1 mg	2 mg	Mild tranquillising dose. Tab. 2 mg, 5 mg, 10 mg. Syrup.
	Oral	2	250 microg/kg		2·5 mg	5 mg	10 mg	Spasmolytic/severe anxiety/pre-med dose.
	I.V.	Single	300 microg/kg					Doses for status epilepticus. Titrate according to response. Caution—transient respiratory distress. Should not be mixed with any other drug. Precipitation may occur in syringe/line—change line six-hourly. See page 123.
	I.V.	Continuous	50 microg/kg/hour					
Diazoxide	Oral	2 or 3	—	5–20 mg/kg/day			100 mg	Coated Tabs. 50 mg. Dose for hypoglycaemia.
	I.V. only	up to 4	—	5 mg/kg			300 mg	Antihypertensive dose.
Dichloralphenazone	Oral	Once	45 mg/kg		450 mg	650 mg	1·3 g	Tabs. 650 mg. Syrup. 225 mg in 5 ml.
Dicyclomine	Oral	3 or 4	—	0·5 mg/kg	5 mg	10 mg	20 mg	Tabs. 10 mg. Syrup.
Digoxin	Oral I.M.	1 or 2	10 microg/kg/day					Once-daily dosing should be adequate. No need for "digitalisation". See page 142. I.V. dose where essential—half stated dose. Elixir 50 microg in 1 ml. Tabs. 62·5 microg, 125 microg, 250 microg. Inj. 100 microg in 1 ml, 500 microg in 2 ml.
Dihydrocodeine bitartrate	Oral	3 or 4	not recommended under 7 years			500 microg/kg	30–60 mg	Tabs. 30 mg. Syrup. Analgesic dose.
	I.M.	as required	not recommended under 7 years			500 microg/kg	50 mg	

Drug	Route	Frequency	Dose/kg				Notes
Dioctyl sodium sulphosuccinate	Oral	3	—	—	5 mg	10 mg	20 mg	As enema 1 mg/kg. Tabs. 20 mg. Syrup.
Droperidol	I.V. I.M. } Oral	Once	300 microg/kg / 100 microg/kg	3·75 mg	7·5 mg	15 mg	Produces "detachment" pre-neurosurgery. Normal premedication dose. Tabs. 2·5 mg, 10 mg.
Edrophonium	I.V.	Single	0·25 mg/kg	1·25 mg	2·5 mg	5 mg	Test for myasthenia gravis. Give 1/5 dose initially. Remainder slowly if tolerated.
Ephedrine	Oral	3	0·8 mg/kg	7·5 mg	15 mg	30 mg	Tabs. 30, 15 and 7·5 mg. Elixir B.P.C. 15 mg/5 ml.
Ethosuximide	Oral	Once	—	125 mg	250 mg	500 mg	Caps. 250 mg. Syrup. See page 207. Therapeutic range—280–700 micromoles/l
Ferrous sulphate	Oral	3	6 mg/kg	60 mg	120 mg	200 mg	Tab. Ferr. Sulph. Co = 200 mg. Paed. Mixt. BNF = 60 mg/5 ml = 12 mg Fe^{++} = 0·2 mmol Fe^{++}.
Folic acid	Oral	Once	—	2·5 mg	5 mg	10 mg	Tabs. 100 microg, 500 microg, and 5 mg.
Frusemide	Oral / I.M. / I.V.	Alt. days or once daily	1–4 mg/kg/day	20 mg (give half oral dose)	40 mg (give quarter oral dose)	40–80 mg	Action complete in 3–4 hours. Tabs. 20 mg. Scored tabs. 40 mg. Liquid.
Glucagon	I.M. / I.V. / S.C.	Once	20 microg/kg	250 microg	500 microg	1 mg	Hypoglycaemia. Diagnostic test in glycogen storage disease.
Haloperidol	Oral	2	25 microg/kg	200 microg	400 microg	1 mg	Liquid 2 mg/ml. Tabs. 1·5 mg. Caps. 0·5 mg. Dose may need to be doubled for "tics".
Heparin	I.V.	—	150 units/kg	2500 units	5000 units	10,000 units	Repeat 4–6 hourly by continuous infusion to maintain the thrombin time or whole-blood clotting time at 2–4 × the control value. Antidote—Protamine sulphate. N.B. The indications for heparin therapy are few. SEEK ADVICE as more appropriate therapy may be available.

SOME IMPORTANT DRUGS—(continued)

Drug	Route	Times Daily	DOSE. Caution. Suggested dose is single dose unless otherwise stated					Availability and Remarks
			0-2/52 Neonatal	2/52-1 year	1 year	7 years	14 plus	
Hydralazine	Oral / I.V.	4 / 4	—	—	From 1 yr. 200 microg/kg Max. 200 mg/day			Tab. 25 mg. 50 mg. Unstable in liquid. For hypertensive crises.
1α-Hydroxy-cholecalciferol	Oral	Once	—	15 nanog/kg				Caps. 250 nanog. 1 microg. Monitor phosphate levels to maintain below 1·9 millimoles/l.
Hyoscine hydrobromide	S.C.	Single	15 microg/kg		150 microg	300 microg	600 microg	Premedication dose.
Imipramine	Oral	3	—	—	—	10 mg	25 mg	Antidepressant dose—may be doubled.
	Oral	ONCE at night	—	—	—	10-25 mg may need 50-75 mg		Nocturnal enuresis dose. Tab. 10 mg and 25 mg. Syrup.
Indomethacin	Oral	—	—	—	—	25 mg b.d.	25 mg t.d.s.	Caps. 25 mg. Suspension. Anti-inflammatory dose.
	Rectal	—	—	—	25 mg	50 mg	100 mg	Supps. 100 mg.
Ipecacuanha	Oral	Single	0-12 mths. 5 ml. 1-2 yrs. 10 ml. Over 2 yrs. 15 ml.					Ipecacuanha Paed. Emetic Draught BPC. See BNF No. 2, 1981, page 353. Follow dose with 200 ml water.
Ketamine	I.V. / I.M.	Single / Single	— / —	2 mg/kg 8-12 mg/kg				Must use a drying agent, e.g. atropine. Do not disturb during recovery.
Lactulose	Oral	2	—	2·5 ml	5 ml	10 ml	15 ml	Dose for constipation.
Magnesium chloride MgCl₂.6H₂O	Oral	3 or 4	0·15 mmol/kg (30 mg/kg) in neonatal hypomagnesaemia according to response.					
Magnesium sulphate MgSO₄.7H₂O	I.M. / I.V.	Once	0·15 mmol/kg (0·075 ml/kg 50% Inj.) in neonatal hypomagnesaemia according to response.					Give. I.V. slowly.

Drug	Route	Frequency	Dose/kg				Notes
Mannitol	I.V.	—	7 ml/kg of a 20% solution I.V. slowly over 30 minutes				Dose for cerebral oedema, see page 124.
			3·5 ml/kg of a 20% solution I.V. slowly over 5 minutes				Dose for renal failure, see page 133. Check no crystallisation of solution.
Mercaptopurine	Oral		For leukaemia see page 172.				Tabs. 50 mg. 10 mg.
Methotrexate	Oral		For leukaemia see page 172.				Tabs. 2·5 mg. 10 mg.
Methylcellulose	Oral	Twice	—	500 mg	1 g	2 g	Granules 2 g = 1 level 5 ml tsp. Tabs. 500 mg. Both followed by water.
Methyldopa	Oral	3	6 mg/kg	62·5 mg	125 mg	250 mg	Increase according to response. Not exceeding 4 times initial dose. Tabs. 125 mg. 250 mg. 500 mg.
Methylphenidate HCl	Oral	2	—	1·25 mg	2·5 mg	5 mg	For hyperkinesia. Adjust dose according to response. Tabs. 10 mg.
Metoclopramide	Oral I.M. I.V.	3 / —	0·1 mg/kg / —	1 mg / 1 mg	5 mg / 5 mg	10 mg / 10 mg	Tabs. 10 mg. Syrup and Paediatric Liquid. Normal therapeutic dose.
Morphine sulph.	I.M. S.C.	3 / —	0·2 mg/kg / 0·15 mg/kg N.B. Avoid if possible	2 mg	4 mg	8–16 mg	Young children show increased susceptibility to resp. depression. Antidote—Naloxone.
Naloxone HCl	I.V. or I.M.	Single Single	10 microg/kg 60 microg/kg				Narcan neonatal 20 microg/ml. See Page 80. Inj. 400 microg/ml.
Neostigmine methyl. sulph.	I.M. I.V.	Once	60 microg/kg	625 microg	1·25 mg	2·5 mg	Atropine usually given first.
Nitrazepam	Oral	2	250 microg/kg	2·5 mg	5 mg	10 mg	Anticonvulsant dose. Tabs. 5 mg.
Pancreatin B.P. 1973	Oral	Total daily dose stated	500 mg/kg	5 g	10 g	20 g	Adjust according to response. Before or with feeds.

SOME IMPORTANT DRUGS—(continued)

Drug	Route	Times Daily	DOSE Caution. Suggested dose is single dose unless otherwise stated					Availability and Remarks
			0-2/52 Neonatal	2/52-1 year	1 year	7 years	14 plus	
Papaveretum	S.C. or I.M.	3	—	0.2 mg/kg	2 mg	5 mg	10-15 mg	
Paracetamol	Oral	4-6 hourly	—	12 mg/kg	120-240 mg	250-500 mg	1 g	Tabs. 500 mg. Elixir Paracetamol for infants B.P.C. contains 120 mg in 5 ml.
Paraldehyde	I.M.	Single	0.1 ml/kg	—	1 ml/yr up to 5 years plus 0.5 ml for each additional year to maximum of 10 ml		10 ml	Deep I.M. Doses above 5 ml divide between sites. Safe to use modern plastic syringes if given within 10 minutes.
Penicillamine	Oral	Once	—	—	2.5 mg-5 mg/kg		250 mg	Dose for rheumatoid arthritis. Tab. 50 mg, 125 mg and 250 mg. Regular blood counts and urine analysis.
Pentamidine	I.M.	Daily	—	See page 263				For Pneumocystitis carinii plus Pyrimethamine.
Pentazocine	Oral	4	—	—		25 mg	50 mg	Tabs. 25 mg. Caps 50 mg Inj.
	I.M.	when required	—		1 mg/kg		30-60 mg	
	I.V.		—		500 microg/kg		30-60 mg	
Pethidine	Oral I.M.	3	1 mg/kg	—	12.5 mg	25 mg	50 mg	Tabs. 25 mg and 50 mg.
Phenobarbitone	Oral I.M.	Once	6 mg/kg as neonatal anticonvulsant, see page 92		30-60 mg	60-90 mg		Anticonvulsant dose. Tab. 15 mg, 30 mg and 60 mg. Elixir. Therapeutic range 40-105 micromoles/l. Paradoxical hyperkinetic effect can occur. For interaction see page 232.
	I.V.	Single	10 mg/kg		8 mg/kg			Dose for status epilepticus. Titrate according to response. Caution—transient respiratory depression. See page 123.

Drug	Route	Doses/day	100 microg/kg	30 microg/kg			Notes
				1 mg	2 mg	4 mg	
Phenoperidine	I.M. or S.C.	3	—	—	—	—	Analgesic dose. I.V. dose is ⅓ stated dose. Resp. depressant dose. For patients on respirators only.
	I.M. or S.C.	Single	—				
Phenytoin	Oral	2	—	5 mg/kg	2–5 mg/kg		Tab. 50 mg and 100 mg. Cap. 25 mg, 50 mg, 100 mg. Susp. 30 mg/5 ml. Therapeutic range 20–100 micromoles/l.
	I.V.	Single		10–15 mg/kg		250 mg	Dose for status epilepticus. Give slowly preferably under ECG control.
Pholcodine	Oral or I.M.	3 or 4	0·1 mg/kg	1 mg	2 mg	5 mg	Pholcodine Linctus, Strong B.P.C. contains 10 mg/5 ml. Pholcodine Linctus B.P.C. contains 5 mg/5 ml.
Phytomenadione (vit. K_1)	Oral or I.M.	—	0·3 mg/kg	3 mg	5 mg	10 mg	Inj. 10 mg or 1 mg.
Potassium chloride	Oral	2 or 3	0·5–1 mmol/kg	6·5 mmol	1 g / 13 mmol	2 g / 26 mmol	Eff. Tab. 500 mg. Liq. 1 mmol/ml. 1 g KCl = 13 mmol.K^+ I.V. Maintenance see pages 56, 81. Better given outside times of a diuretic's effect.
Pot. effervescent Tabs. B.P.C. 1 Tab. = 6·5 mmol K^+	Oral	3		1 Tab.	2 Tabs.	4 Tabs.	n.b. This palatable alternative does not contain any chloride.
Prochlorperazine	Oral	3		1·25–2·5 mg	5 mg	5–10 mg	Antiemetic dose stated. Tab. 5 mg, 25 mg. Syrup.
	I.M.	Single		1·25 mg	3·125 mg–6·25 mg	12·5 mg	May be used up to 8-hourly if necessary when receiving cytotoxic therapy.
	Rectal	Single		2·5 mg	5–10 mg	12·5–25 mg	Suppos. 5 mg, 25 mg.
Procyclidine	Oral	3		—	1·25 mg	2·5 mg	Anti-Parkinson effect. Adjust dose according to response. Tabs. 5 mg.
Promethazine HCl	Oral	3	1·5 mg/kg	15 mg	25 mg	25–50 mg	Tabs. 10 mg, 25 mg. Syrup 5 mg/5 ml.

SOME IMPORTANT DRUGS—(continued)

Drug	Route	Times Daily	DOSE Caution. Suggested dose is single dose unless otherwise stated					Availability and Remarks
			0-2/52 Neonatal	2/52-1 year	1 year	7 years	14 plus	
Propranolol	Oral	2 or 3	—	1 mg/kg	10 mg	20 mg	40 mg	Tabs. 10 mg, 40 mg, 80 mg. Adjust dose. As prophylaxis in migraine use half stated dose.
Protamine sulph.	I.V.	—	Slowly 1 mg (0.1 ml) for each 100 units Heparin to maximum of 50 mg.					Inj. 10 mg/ml.
Salbutamol	Oral	3 or 4	—	100 microg/kg	1 mg	2 mg	4 mg	Tabs. 2 mg, 4 mg, 8 mg (long-acting) and Syrup. N.B. Inj. is available.
	Metered Inhal.	3 or 4	—	—	—	100 microg	100-200 microg	100 microg/metered dose.
	Inhal.	3 or 4	—	—	—	200 microg	200-400 microg	"Rotacaps" 200 microg and 400 microg.
	Nebul.	3 or 4	—	—	2.5 mg	5 mg	—	Resp. Soln. 5 mg/ml. Dilute dose to 2 ml with 0.9% Na.Cl. May increase up to 8 times/day.
Senna standardised	Oral	Once at night	—	—	7.5 mg	15 mg	30 mg	Dose expressed as total sennosides. 7.5 mg=1 tablet=5 ml syrup.
Sodium aurothiomalate	I.M.	Weekly	—	—	—	10 mg	25-50 mg	Response may not be apparent until 12 inj. given. Weekly inj. and if tolerated and effective, maintain with the monthly inj. Regular blood counts and urine analysis. Watch for side-effects.
Sodium cromoglycate	Inhal. Orally	3	—	—	—	20 mg	20-40 mg	"Spincaps" 20 mg.
	Nebuliser	3	—	—	10-20 mg	—	—	Nebuliser soln. 20 mg/2 ml.
	Nasal	4	—	—	—	10 mg/nostril	—	Insufflator cap. 10 mg.
	Nasal	6	—	—	one dose/nostril	2 doses/nostril		Metered spray. Nasal drops and spray.

Drug	Route	Doses			10–25 mg/kg	400 mg	800 mg	Notes
Sodium valproate	Oral	2	—	—	10–25 mg/kg	400 mg	800 mg	Tab. 200 mg, 200 mg E/C, 500 mg E/C, 500 mg E/C. Syrup 200 mg in 5 ml.
Spironolactone	Oral	2	—	1·2 mg/kg	12·5 mg	25 mg	50 mg	Tab. 25 mg scored and 100 mg. Double dose may be given once per day.
Sulphasalazine	Oral	4	—	—	250 mg	500 mg	1 g	Ulcerative Colitis. Tab. 500 mg.
Terbutaline	Oral	3	—	150 microg/kg	1·5 mg	5 mg	5 mg	Tab. 5 mg and Syrup.
	Metered	1 or 2	—	—	—	250 microg	250–500 microg	250 microg/metered dose, or by "spacer" inhaler.
	Nebul.	3 or 4	—	—	2 mg	2–5 mg	—	Resp. soln. 10 mg/ml. Dilute dose to 2 ml with 0·9% NaCl. N.B. Inj. is available.
Theophylline, its salts and derivatives:								
(1) Aminophylline	Oral	2	For use in preterm apnoea, page 86.			100 mg daily ↓ 225 mg b.d.	225 mg b.d. ↓ 450 mg b.d.	"Phyllocontin" dosage given. Sust. release tab. 100 mg, 225 mg. Start low and increase dose slowly.
	I.V.				4 mg/kg initially slowly over 10 minutes, then 0·7 mg/kg/hour. maximum 20 mg/kg/24 hours.			I.V. inj. 250 mg in 10 ml. See page 129.
(2) Choline theophyllinate	Oral	3 or 4	—		5–8 mg/kg/dose max. 32 mg/kg/day		200 mg	Tab. 100 mg and 200 mg. Syrup 62·5 mg in 5 ml.
(3) Theophylline	Oral	3 or 4	—		5 mg/kg/dose as Theophylline		250 mg	"Nuelin" dose given. Tabl. 125 mg. Liquid contain 60 mg theophylline hyd. (= 120 mg theophylline glycinate) in 5 ml.
	Oral	2	—			175 mg	250 mg	"Nuelin S.A." dose given. S.A. Tab. 175 mg. 250 mg.
	Oral	2	—		10–12 mg/kg/dose	125–250 mg	250–500 mg	"Rona-Slophyllin" dose given. Sust. release Cap. 60 mg, 125 mg, 250 mg.
			For all Theophylline preparations established therapeutic range is 55–110 micromoles/l of Theophylline.					Above dose variation due to different commercially available preparations.

SOME IMPORTANT DRUGS—(continued)

Drug	Route	Times Daily	DOSE Caution. Suggested dose is single dose unless otherwise stated					Availability and Remarks
			0-2/52 Neonatal	2/52- 1 year	1 year	7 years	14 plus	
Thyroxine	Oral	Once	12·5 microg		25 microg	50 microg	100 microg	Initial dose stated. Increase dose at 2/52 intervals according to response. Tab. 25 microg, 50 microg, 100 microg.
Tranexamic acid	Oral	3	—		30 mg/kg			Contra-indicated in renal impairment, haematuria etc. Tab. 500 mg.
	I.V.	No more than 8-hrly	—		15 mg/kg by slow I.V. infusion over at least 10 minutes.			DO NOT mix I.V. with penicillins or blood.
Trimeprazine tart.	Oral	3	—	250 microg/kg	2·5 mg	5 mg	10 mg	Antipruritic dose. Tab. 10 mg and syrup.
	Oral	Single	—	3 mg/kg			—	Pre-med dose.
Vincristine	I.V.		For leukaemia see page 172.					
Warfarin	Oral	Once	—	First day 0·75 mg/kg	7·5 mg	15 mg	27 mg	Loading dose guidelines stated—seek haematological advice. Decrease dose if liver function impaired. Tabs. 1 mg, 3 mg and 5 mg.
				Second day No treatment.				
				Thereafter according to Prothrombin time or "Thrombotest". Daily maintenance dose is approximately 1/5 of loading dose.				

N.M.D.
G.R.

[NOTES]

[NOTES]

[NOTES]

[NOTES]

XII
ANTIMICROBIAL AGENTS

GENERAL CONSIDERATIONS

Before antimicrobial therapy is started, appropriate specimens, such as CSF, blood culture, pus, urine, etc., should be obtained, in order that the causative microbe can be identified and its antimicrobial sensitivity determined.

In the ill child a suitable antimicrobial agent or combination should be given, based on the likely pathogens in the condition, pending laboratory results. When limited laboratory results are available, e.g. microscopic identification of pathogens in CSF, therapy may be tailored to that organism. In other situations, however, e.g. wound infection following large-bowel surgery, several organisms, including anaerobic, may be involved, and therapy should take these into account.

Those antimicrobial agents which are used in life-threatening infections, e.g. gentamicin and sodium fusidate, should be reserved for such use and not used topically.

Tetracyclines should not be used in children except topically. They cause tooth staining in children without permanent dentition, and alternative agents are available.

Route

The oral route is contra-indicated by vomiting or diarrhoea or when therapeutic blood levels are needed rapidly, although parenteral therapy is less practical than the oral route in outpatients. When a combination of drugs by the parenteral route is indicated, each drug should be administered separately. Where one antimicrobial agent is to be given three times daily and another four, it may be simpler to adjust the individual dosage size and administer both drugs at the same frequency.

Choice of Agent

Initial choice for particular infections will be influenced by local antimicrobial policies and antimicrobial resistance patterns. Several effective regimens are available for many infections.

Suggested initial therapy:
Meningitis.

Neonatal	Chloramphenicol *or* benzylpenicillin plus gentamicin.
Other ages (blind treatment).	Sulphadimidine plus benzylpenicillin plus chloramphenicol.
Haemophilus.	Chloramphenicol.
Pneumococcus.	Benzylpenicillin.
Meningococcus.	Benzylpenicillin (and sulphadimidine to eradicate nasopharyngeal carriage).
Listeria.	Ampicillin and gentamicin.

N.B. Many antimicrobials including penicillins, cephalosporins and aminoglycosides cross the blood-brain barrier poorly. The choice is determined by both the sensitivity of the organism and the need to achieve adequate levels across the blood-brain barrier.

Acute Osteomyelitis/ Septic Arthritis.	Flucloxacillin plus fusidic acid/ sodium fusidate.
Infective Endocarditis.	Benzylpenicillin plus gentamicin. Dosage control in co-operation with microbiologist.
Peritonitis.	Metronidazole plus cefuroxime (or cefoxitin).
Cellulitis.	Flucloxacillin.
Pneumonia.	Lobar:—Benzylpenicillin. Bronchopneumonia, hospital acquired:—Ampicillin plus gentamicin Bronchopneumonia, not hospital acquired—Ampicillin plus flucloxacillin.
Acute Epiglottitis.	Chloramphenicol.
Diphtheria.	Contact microbiologist if suspected. Benzylpenicillin and antitoxin.
Acute Otitis.	Co-trimoxazole or ampicillin/amoxycillin.
Acute Lower Urinary Tract Infection.	Trimethoprim alone or co-trimoxazole or ampicillin/amoxycillin.

Suspected Pyelonephritis (loin pain).	Co-trimoxazole (ampicillin parenteral therapy for vomiting patient).
Neonatal Conjunctivitis.	Neomycin topically. If not improving after 24 hours suspect: Chlamydia—Topical tetracycline plus oral erythromycin Gonococci—Topical plus parenteral benzylpenicillin.
Septicaemia.	Treat appropriately, based on infective focus as above. If no apparent focus treat with benzylpenicillin, gentamicin plus metronidazole.

Antimicrobial Side-Effects

During normal course of therapy	Gastro-intestinal:
	(1) Diarrhoea (common)
	(2) Candida
	(3) Staphylococcal overgrowth (uncommon)
	(4) Pseudomembraneous colitis (rare).
	Rashes.
	Fever:
	Thrombophlebitis from I.V. therapy.
	Sulphonamides and ampicillin during treatment of meningitis.
	Renal toxicity:
	Sulphonamides (crystalluria)
	Polymyxins, aminoglycosides especially when combined with diuretics or certain cephalosporins.
Variable time after stopping therapy	Blood dyscrasias:
	Chloramphenicol
	Ototoxicity:
	Gentamicin, tobramycin.
	Neomycin inhalations.

Prophylaxis

Widespread prophylaxis should be avoided. Recognised indications for antimicrobial prophylaxis are:

(1) Prevention of recurrent urinary tract infections.
(2) Prevention of further rheumatic fever below age 18 years.
(3) Splenectomised patients and sickle-cell disease (pneumococcal infection).
(4) Prevention of endocarditis (known valve lesion) following dental extraction, urinary catheterisation and other procedures likely to produce bacteraemia.
(5) Family contacts of meningococcal infection (sulphadimidine if strain sensitive).
(6) Neonate exposed to TB—isoniazid plus INAH resistant BCG.
(7) Certain surgical operations, e.g. large-bowel surgery, when there is an appreciable risk of infection. Therapy should achieve maximal blood levels at time of operation and should be discontinued after 24 hours.
(8) Suspected *Bordetella pertussis* contact in unvaccinated child—erythromycin to all children, especially infants under 1 year.

ANTIMICROBIAL AGENTS—ANTIBIOTICS

Drug	Route	Times Daily	DOSE — Caution. Suggested dose is single dose unless otherwise stated					Availability and Remarks
			0-2/52 Neonatal	2/52-1 year	1 year	7 years	14 plus	
Amoxycillin	Oral	3	62.5 mg		125 mg	250 mg	500 mg	Cap. 250 mg and Syrup. Inj. also available.
Ampicillin	Oral I.M. I.V.	4	see page 94	62.5 mg	125 mg	250 mg	500 mg	Meningitis dose = 400 mg/kg/day by continuous I.V. for 10 days. Tabs. 125 mg. Caps. 250 mg. Syrup.
Carbenicillin	I.M. I.V.	4	see page 94	50 mg/kg	500 mg	1 g	2 g	Dose may be quadrupled I.V. in severe infections. Use concurrently with Probenecid.
Cefoxitin	I.M. I.V.	3	—	—	25-50 mg/kg		2 g	Adjust in significant renal impairment. Preferable to use I.V. route.
Cefuroxime	I.M. I.V.	3	30 mg/kg 12-hourly see page 94	30 mg/kg	250 mg	500 mg	1 g	Dose for severe infections. Adjust in significant renal impairment.
Cephazolin	I.M. I.V.	4	—	25 mg/kg	250 mg	500 mg	1 g	Adjust in significant renal impairment.
Cephalexin	Oral	4	12 mg/kg		125 mg	250 mg	500 mg	Caps. 250 mg and 500 mg. Susp.
Chloramphenicol	Oral	4	Avoid	12 mg/kg	125 mg	250 mg	500 mg	Dose for typhoid Cap. 250 mg. Syrup.
	I.V.	4	See page 94		25 mg/kg			Dose for meningitis Assess blood levels—maintain peak 15-25 mg/l. I.T. dose 1-2 mg daily. For interactions see page 232
Clindamycin	Oral	3 or 4	—	37.5 mg	75 mg	150 mg	300 mg	Caps. 75 mg and 150 mg. Susp.
	I.M. I.V.	4	—	5-10 mg/kg			300-600 mg	I.V. as infusion over 30 minutes.

ANTIMICROBIAL AGENTS—ANTIBIOTICS—*(continued)*

Drug	Route	Times Daily	0-2/52 Neonatal	2/52-1 year	1 year	7 years	14 plus	Availability and Remarks
Co-trimoxazole	Oral	2	Avoid	4 mg/kg	40 mg	80 mg	160 mg	Doses stated in terms of Trimethoprim. Prophylaxis: half stated dose at night.
	I.M.	2	Avoid	—	—	3 mg/kg	160 mg	I.M. not recommended under 6 years.
	I.V.	2	Avoid	3 mg/kg			160 mg	I.V. as infusion over 1 hour. Adjust in renal impairment.
	Oral I.V. }	2	Avoid	10 mg/kg				Dose for *Pneumocystis carinii*—treat for 14 days.
Erythromycin	Oral	4	12·5 mg/kg		125 mg	250 mg	500 mg	Tab. 250 mg, 500 mg. Cap. 250 mg. Susp. See literature for suitable salts for long-term use (beware jaundice).
	I.M.	3	2·5 mg/kg		25 mg	50 mg	100 mg	Preferable to give I.V. as below. Special I.M. inj.
	I.V.	4	8-12 mg/kg			300 mg	300-600 mg	Special I.V. inj.
Ethambutol	Oral	Once	—		15 mg/kg			Caution in renal impairment. 25 mg/kg for retreatment. Tabs. 100 mg, 400 mg.
Flucloxacillin and Cloxacillin	Oral I.M. or I.V.	4	see page 94	62·5 mg	125 mg	250 mg	500 mg	Flucloxacillin better absorbed orally. Caps. 250 mg. Syrup. Adult I/T dose 10 mg. Dose for severe infection.
Fusidic Acid	Oral	4	—	12·5 mg/kg as Acid		250 mg Sod.	500 mg Sod.	Cap. 250 mg. (Sod. salt.) Susp. 250 mg (Acid) in 5 ml.
	I.V.	3	Give as diethanolamine fusidate, 6-7 mg /kg/8-hourly (≦ 5 mg sodium fusidate). For *severe* infections the dose may be doubled.				500 mg	
Gentamicin	I.M. I.V.	3	see page 94	2·5 mg/kg				Assess blood levels—maintain peak levels below 12 mg/l; trough levels below 2 mg/l. Adjust dose in renal impairment. I.V. by bolus inj. ONLY. I.T. dose 1-2 mg.

			10–15 mg/kg	100 mg	200 mg	300 mg	
Isoniazid (I.N.A.H.)	Oral	Once	—	10 mg/kg		300 mg	Tab. 50 mg and 100 mg. Pyridoxine may be given concurrently.
	I.M. I.V.	Once					Initially in TB Meningitis.
Metronidazole	Oral	3	7–8 mg/kg 12-hourly	7–8 mg/kg		400 mg	Treatment dose for Bacteroides. Tab. 200 mg and 400 mg. Susp.
	I.V.	3	7–8 mg/kg 12-hourly	7–8 mg/kg		500 mg	Inj. to be protected from light. Neonatal dose see page 94.
	Rectal	3	—	125 mg	500 mg	1 g	Suppos. 500 mg and 1 g. For antiparasitic use see page 111.
Nalidixic acid	Oral	4	Avoid	250 mg	500 mg	1 g	Tabs. 500 mg. Suspension.
Neomycin	Oral	4	12 mg/kg	125 mg	250 mg	500 mg	Not absorbed. Tabs. 500 mg. Syrup.
Nitrofurantoin	Oral	4 night	2·5 mg/kg 2·5 mg/kg	25 mg 25 mg	50 mg 50 mg	100 mg 100 mg	Tabs. 50 mg and 100 mg. Suspension. For Prophylaxis.
Penicillin G.	I.M.	4	see page 94 — 15 mg/kg	150 mg (¼ mega)	300 mg (½ mega)	600 mg (1 mega)	Crystalline or Benzyl Penicillin 1 mega unit = 600 mg.
	I.V.	4 to 6	25–50 mg/kg				For severe infections by bolus inj. ONLY over 5 minutes.
	I.T.	Once	0·3 mg	2–5 mg			Never above 5 mg in a child under 12.
Penicillin prolonged action	I.M. only	—	¼ vial	½ vial		1 vial	Each vial contains: Penicillin G. 300 mg. Procaine Pen. 250 mg. Benethamine Pen. 475 mg.
Penicillin V. Phenoxymethyl Penicillin	Oral	4	62·5 mg	125 mg	250 mg	500 mg	Tabs. 125 mg and 250 mg. Syrup.
Rifampicin	Oral	Daily	— 15–20 mg/kg (maximum 600 mg dose)			600 mg	Caps. 150 mg and 300 mg. Susp. 100 mg in 5 ml. Caution with impaired liver function.
	Oral	Daily	— 10–20 mg/kg			600 mg	Daily for 4 days for meningoccocal carriers.

ANTIMICROBIAL AGENTS—ANTIBIOTICS—(continued)

Drug	Route	Times Daily	DOSE Caution. Suggested dose is single dose unless otherwise stated					Availability and Remarks
			0-2/52 Neonatal	2/52- 1 year	1 year	7 years	14 plus	
Streptomycin	I.M.	Once	Avoid	25 mg/kg	250 mg	500 mg	1 g	Occasionally indicated in TB.
Sulphadimidine	Oral I.V.	4	Avoid	25 mg/kg	250 mg	500 mg	1 g	Dose doubled in severe infection. Tabs. 500 mg. Mixture 500 mg/5ml.
Tetracycline HCl. and Oxytetracycline			Not recommended in children except topically					
Tobramycin	I.M.	3	3 mg/kg 12-hourly	2·5 mg/kg				Assess blood levels—maintain peak levels below 12 mg/l; trough levels below 2 mg/l. Adjust dose in renal impairment. I.V. by bolus inj. ONLY.
Trimethoprim	Oral	2	—	4mg/kg	50 mg	100 mg	200 mg	Dose for treatment Tab. 100 mg. Susp.

ANTIMICROBIAL AGENTS—ANTIFUNGALS

Drug	Route	Times Daily	DOSE Caution. Suggested dose is single dose unless otherwise stated					Availability and Remarks
			0-2/52 Neonatal	2/52-1 year	1 year	7 years	14 plus	
Amphotericin B.	I.V.		—	250 units/kg administered by slow intravenous infusion over a period of 6 hours.	2500 units	5000 units	10,000 units	Initial dose stated. Increase gradually up to maximum of 4×stated dose, depending on toxicity. Given every 2 days. N.B. Special diluent.
	Oral		50–100 mg after each feed.					Oral thrush. Tab. 100 mg. Susp. 100 mg/ml. Lozenges 10 mg.
Flucytosine	Oral I.V.	4	50 mg/kg 12-hrly.	50 mg/kg				Tab. 500 mg scored. Adjust dose in renal impairment. I.V. Infusion over 30 minutes. N.B. Special storage required for inj.
Griseofulvin	Oral	2	—		5 mg/kg		500 mg once	Tab. 125 mg and 500 mg. Susp.
Miconazole	Oral	4	62·5 mg b.d.	125 mg b.d.	125 mg	125 mg	250 mg	Tab. 250 mg. Oral gel 125 mg/5 ml. Little oral absorption.
	I.V.	3	—	12–15 mg/kg			600 mg	I.V. infusion over at least 30 minutes
Nystatin	Oral		Oral thrush 100,000 units on tongue after each feed.					Oral susp. and Tab. ½ mega. Little absorption.

ANTIMICROBIAL AGENTS—ANTIPARASITICS

Drug	Route	Times Daily	DOSE Caution. Suggested dose is single dose unless otherwise stated					Availability and Remarks
			0-2/52 Neonatal	2/52-1 year	1 year	7 years	14 plus	
Bephenium	Oral	Once	—	2·5 g Give on empty stomach and no food for 1 hour after dose.			5 g	Sachets 5 g. Hookworm (Ancylostomiasis) and Roundworms (Ascariasis). See page 110.
Chloroquine as base	Oral	Once	—	10 mg/kg immediately, then 5 mg/kg after 6 hours, then 5 mg/kg daily for 2 days.				Tab. Chlor. Phos. 250 mg = 150 mg base. Tab. Chlor. Sulph. 200 mg = 150 mg base. Syrup 50 mg base in 5 ml. I.V. given slowly by infusion in inj. Sod. Chloride 0·9%—change to oral therapy as soon as possible. See page 105.
"Maloprim"	Oral	Once weekly	—	—	—	½ tablet	1 tablet	Each tablet contains: Dapsone 100 mg and Pyrimethamine 12·5 mg. See page 106.
Mebendazole	Oral	2	—	—	100 mg 2 years to adults	100 mg		Tab. 100 mg. Susp. Anthelminthic 3-day course. See page 110.
Metronidazole	Oral	Once	—		40 mg/kg	1 g	2 g	Dose for Giardiasis—treat for 3 days.
	Oral	3	—		20 mg/kg	400 mg	800 mg	Dose for Amoebiasis— Invasive—treat for 5 days. Asymptomatic excretors treat for 10 days. See page 111.
Niclosamide	Oral	Single dose	—		500 mg	1 g	2 g	Tab. 500 mg. See pages 110-111. Tapeworm (Taeniasis) half stated dose, then repeat after 1 hour. Purge after 2 hours. H. Nana—stated dose on 1st day, half stated dose for following 6 days.

Drug	Route	Frequency						Notes
					4 mg/kg daily for 10–14 days.			
Pentamidine	I.M.	Daily	—					For *Pneumocystis carinii* plus pyrimethamine. See under Pyrimethamine.
Piperazine	Oral	Once	—	50 mg/kg	750 mg	1·5 g	2 g	Tab. 500 mg. Elixir. See page 110. Enterobius—stated dose daily for 7 days. Ascaris—twice stated dose once in the morning.
Piperazine + Senna	Oral	Once	—	⅓ sachet	⅔ sachet		1 sachet	"Pripsen" sachet contains 4 g Piperazine+Senna. Enterobius & Ascaris—one dose, repeat at 14 days. See page 110.
Primaquine as base	Oral	Daily for 14 days	—	375 microg/kg	3·75 mg	7·5 mg	15 mg	Coated tab. contain 7·5 mg base. Unstable in liq. form. For eradication of *P. vivax* following 3-day course of Chloroquine. See page 106.
Pyrimethamine	Oral	Once	—	—	6·25 mg	12·5 mg	25 mg	Scored tab. 25 mg. Elixir. For Toxoplasmosis 12-day course plus Sulphonamides in full dosage for 28 days with Folinic Acid supplement. For *Pneumocystis carinii* 12-day course with Pentamidine.
Quinine HCl.	I.V.	12-hourly	—	5–10 mg/kg Slow I.V. inf. over 4 hours at conc. 50–100 mg/100 ml				For cerebral malaria. Use the lower dose if fits, etc. occur during therapy. See page 106.
Thiabendazole	Oral	2	—	25 mg/kg	25 mg/kg		1·5 g	Tab. 500 mg. Take with food. See page 110. Enterobius—treat for 1 day and repeat at 7 days. Trichinosis—treat for 4 days. Other worms—treat for 2 days.

N.M.D.
R.H.G.
G.R.

[NOTES]

XIII
CORTICOSTEROIDS

GENERAL CONSIDERATIONS

The dosage of some synthetic steroids in common usage is given on page 269. Side-effects of steroid therapy can be minimised by giving 48 hours' dosage as a single dose on alternate days. Corticotrophin (ACTH) is used when it is necessary to stimulate the patient's adrenal cortex.

PRECAUTIONS IN TREATMENT

Careful watch for signs of infection should be maintained and antibiotic therapy started more readily than usual if infection is suspected. When an infection, or other stress such as a surgical operation, is encountered in a child, the maintenance dose of the drug, if small, should be increased 3 times. When the drug is stopped the adrenal cortex may take some time to recover and, therefore, during the following year any infection should be covered by the equivalent of 50 mg of cortisone daily.

Scheme of steroid cover before, during and after operation

For children who have received steroids in prolonged or heavy dosage, whether oral, systemic or by rectum, at any time during the previous two years the following scheme is suggested. If the daily dose has been more than 100 mg of cortisone or its equivalent, double the amounts pre- and post-operatively, returning to the previous dose on the fourth day.

12 hours before operation:	100 mg cortisone I.M.
1 hour before operation:	100 mg cortisone I.M.
First 24 hours post-operatively:	50 mg cortisone by mouth 6-hourly or 100 mg I.M. 12-hourly.
Second 24 hours post-operatively:	50 mg cortisone 8-hourly by mouth or 75 mg I.M. 12-hourly.
Third 24 hours post-operatively:	50 mg cortisone 12-hourly by mouth or I.M. if necessary.

Fourth 24 hours post-operatively: 25 mg cortisone 12-hourly by mouth or I.M. if necessary.

During operation and for 24 hours afterwards hydrocortisone for intravenous use must be *immediately available* in the theatre or at the bedside.

OUT-PATIENT CARE

Upon discharge from hospital the family doctor and the parents must be instructed that (1) the drug must be taken exactly as prescribed, (2) that the dose must be raised during infection or stress to 3 times the normal daily dose. When the child is on continuous or alternate-day "high dose" treatment, the dose at time of stress need not be higher than that used at the start of treatment.

Parents of children who are non-immune to varicella and measles should be warned of the potential hazards and advised to report any contact immediately so that appropriate protective measures (page 108) can be taken.

A card giving details of therapy should be issued to all patients with advice to carry it at all times.

PRINCIPAL STEROIDS AND INITIAL DOSE

Drug	Route	Times Daily	DOSE Caution. Suggested dose is single dose unless otherwise stated					Availability and Remarks
			0-2/52 Neonatal	2/52-1 year	1 year	7 years	14 plus	
ACTH (Corticotrophin Gel)	I.M.	Once	—	1 i.u./kg	10 i.u.	20 i.u.	40 i.u.	Long-acting.
Tetracosactrin (Synacthen Depot)	I.M.	Once	—	0·25 mg			0·5– 1 mg	Long-acting. ACTH test see page 192.
Beclomethasone	Metered Inhal.	2–4			—	50 microg	100 microg	50 microg per metered dose.
	Inhal.	2–4			—	100 microg	200 microg	"Rotacaps" 100 & 200 microg.
Dexamethasone	I.V.		—	100 microg/kg I.V. immediately then 50 microg/kg. 6-hourly.				Dose for cerebral oedema stated. See page 124.
Fludrocortisone acetate	Oral	Once	—	5 microg/kg	50 microg	100 microg	200 microg	Tab. 100 microg. 1 mg.
Hydrocortisone hemisuccinate	I.V. I.M.		All ages—Pharmacological doses 50–100 mg repeatable 6-hourly.					Dose for status asthmaticus, see page 129.
Methylprednisolone	I.V.		—		15–30 mg/kg			Inj. 40 mg, 125 mg, 500 mg.
Prednisolone and Prednisone	Oral	3		250–500 microg/kg				Tab. 1 mg, 5 mg. Sol. Tabs. 5 mg. } Prednisolone E/C. Tabs. 2·5 mg, 5 mg. } only. Use smallest dose to control symptoms/signs. Reduce before stopping.

Dose for Idiopathic Nephrotic Syndrome 60 mg/m²/day. Max. 80 mg/day, see page 131.

Equivalent (anti-inflammatory) doses of other steroids are shown below. These figures also correspond with tablet strength.

Cortisone	25 mg	Hydrocortisone	20 mg
Dexamethasone	0·75 mg	Prednisone	5 mg
Methylprednisolone	5 mg		

N.M.D.
G.R.

[NOTES]

[NOTES]

[NOTES]

[NOTES]

INDEX

INDEX

intragastric and intrajejunal, 26
sick infants, 25–27
sick newborns, 26, 81
Feeds, *see also* Milk formulae
normal, composition, 24
special composition, 33–40
Fetoscopy, 211
Fits, *see* Convulsions
Fluids, daily needs, 53
diet, formula, 26
and electrolyte therapy, 53–59
insensible loss under heaters, 61, 88
intravenous, 53
Formulae, *see* Milk formulae
Fresh frozen plasma, 96, 169

G-6-PD deficiency, 101, 106, 167
Galactosaemia, 198
Galactose-low diet, 41
Gammaglobulin in virus infections, 98–99, 108, 112, 171
Gangliosidoses, 199
Gastro-enteritis, 25, 117, 203
Gastro-intestinal function tests, 182
Gastro-intestinal symptoms in the newborn, 97
Genetic counselling, 208
Gentamicin, drug level, 258
Giardia lamblia, 111, 183
Glucagon, newborn hypoglycaemia, 84
Glucagon test, 197
Gluten-free diet, 41
Glycogen storage disease, 199
Growth, charts, addresses, 3–4
hormone screening test, 194
insulin sensitivity test, 194
tables, 3–4

Haematological disorders, 163–168
values, 169
Haemoglobinopathies, 165–167
Haemolytic diseases of the newborn, 89
Haemolytic uraemic syndrome, 133
Haemophila, 163
dental extractions, 163
Haemorrhage in the newborn, 95
Haemorrhagic disorders, 163–165
Heart failure, 127, 142
Hepatitis, and P.U.O., 107

and the newborn, 99
Herpes simplex, and P.U.O., 108
and newborn, 99
Homocystinuria, 199
Hormones, 188–192
reference values, 188–192
releasing, 188
trophic, 188
Hydramnios, 77, 96
Hydrocephalus, blocked shunt, 126
Hypernatraemia, 55, 118
Hypertensive crisis, 136
Hypocalcaemia, in the newborn, 90
Hypoglycaemia, in CAH, 122
investigation, 197–198
newborn, 83–84
parenteral nutrition, 67
treatment, 123
Hypomagnesaemia, newborn, 91
Hyponatraemia, 135, 146
and dehydration, 54–56
differential diagnosis, 120
management, 120–122
Hypoproteinaemia, 29, 131

Idiopathic respiratory distress syndrome, 85
Ill baby, the, 92–95
Immunisation, and contra-indications, 112
schedules, 113
for travel, 114
Inborn errors of metabolism, tests for, 198
Incubation periods, 109
Infection in the newborn, 93–95, 98–99
Infectious disease, incubations and isolation, 109
Inquest, advice on attending, 216
Insensible fluid loss, 61, 88, 134
Insulin, assay, 197
dosage, 139
Insulin sensitivity test, 194
Insulins, types and action of, 138
Intravenous fluids, calcium, 58
maintenance therapy, 53
in the newborn, 61, 81
potassium, 56
rehydration, 54
sodium bicarbonate, 57
solutions, 58